S0-BRV-930

Policies and Procedures of a
Cardiac Rehabilitation Program
Immediate to Long-term Care

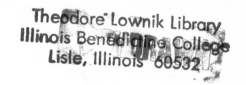
Theodore Lownik Library
Illinois Benedictine College
Lisle, Illinois 60532

Policies and Procedures of a

Cardiac Rehabilitation Program

Immediate to Long-term Care

Philip K. Wilson, Ed.D.

Executive Director, La Crosse Exercise Program, and
Professor, Physical Education Department,
School of Health, Physical Education and Recreation,
University of Wisconsin-La Crosse, La Crosse, Wisconsin

Edward R. Winga, M.D.

Gundersen Clinic, Ltd., and La Crosse Lutheran Hospital;
Executive Board, La Crosse Exercise Program, and
Adjunct Faculty, University of Wisconsin-La Crosse, La Crosse, Wisconsin

Joseph W. Edgett, M.D.

Gundersen Clinic, Ltd., and La Crosse Lutheran Hospital;
Executive Board, La Crosse Exercise Program, and
Adjunct Faculty, University of Wisconsin-La Crosse, La Crosse, Wisconsin

Thomas T. Gushiken, Ph.D.

Unit Director, Workshop Unit, La Crosse Exercise Program, and
Assistant Professor, Recreation and Parks Department,
School of Health, Physical Education and Recreation,
University of Wisconsin-La Crosse, La Crosse, Wisconsin

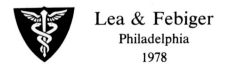
Lea & Febiger
Philadelphia
1978

362
.1961
P766

Library of Congress Cataloging in Publication Data

Main entry under title:

Policies and procedures of a cardiac rehabilitation program.

Bibliography: p.
Includes index.
1. Cardiovascular patient—Rehabilitation—Planning.
2. Community health services—Administration.
3. Community health services—Wisconsin—La Crosse—
Administration. I. Wilson, Philip K. [DNLM:
1. Heart diseases—Rehabilitation. WG200.3 P766]
RC682.P64   362.1'9'6106   78-5899.
ISBN 0-8121-0635-0

Copyright © 1978 by Lea & Febiger. Copyright under the International Copyright
Union. All rights reserved. This book is protected by copyright. *No part of it may be
reproduced in any manner or by any means without written permission from the
publisher.*

Published in Great Britain by Henry Kimpton Publishers, London

PRINTED IN THE UNITED STATES OF AMERICA

Print No.   3   2   1

Preface

The benefits of regular exercise to accomplish optimum individual levels of physical fitness has received such notoriety in the popular press that one would think the benefits of exercise has been a recently discovered phenomenon. Suddenly we see thousands of people jogging through our cities and towns, and those who aren't jogging seem to be cycling, swimming, playing tennis, or participating in other forms of vigorous physical activity. Bookstores are deluged with titles telling the lay person "how to" run, swim, cycle, jump rope, play tennis, and perform many other types of physical exercise. It does appear that at long last the American public has come to realize that physiological benefits of optimal health may be obtained through regular vigorous physical exercise.

That the lack of exercise might contribute to our population's high rate of coronary artery disease has been suspected for many years and studied by many scientists. To "counterattack" the "heart attack" and to provide a mechanism of recovery for the cardiac surgery patient through a program of progressive exercise is the goal of the Cardiac Rehabilitation Program of La Crosse, Wisconsin. The La Crosse Cardiac Rehabilitation Program is conducted under strictly defined guidelines, with the gradually progressing exercise of the patient dependent upon data provided from graded exercise testing and related laboratory measurements. A program of cardiac rehabilitation must incorporate safeguards and procedures that prevent the individual from overexertion and provide immediate means of handling any emergency that might arise despite these precautions.

The establishment of a cardiac rehabilitation program requires great attention to organizational and administrative details. The La Crosse Cardiac Rehabilitation Program has been in operation since early 1971. It is a "total" program, developed through the efforts of the personnel and services of Gundersen Clinic Ltd., La Crosse Lutheran Hospital, and the School of Health, Physical Education, and Recreation of the University of Wisconsin-La Crosse. Over the years the program has expanded and grown, and accordingly the policies and procedures of the program have been reexamined, redeveloped, and tested. This book contains policies and procedures which have proven to be successful, providing an efficient and effective program.

We believe that this book will be an essential resource and ready reference for all medical, paramedical, and community service personnel interested in cardiac rehabilitation, and the related topics of graded exercise testing, exercise prescription, and patient education.

Much of the material within this text has been adapted from procedures performed within La Crosse area hospitals and clinics. We express our appreciation to the staff and services of the following institutions and agencies for their continued support to the La Crosse Cardiac Rehabilitation Program:

> Adolph Gundersen Medical Foundation
> Gundersen Clinic, Ltd.
> La Crosse County Medical Society
> La Crosse Lutheran Hospital
> La Crosse Clinic
> Skemp-Grandview Clinic
> St. Francis Hospital
> Wisconsin Heart Association

> Philip K. Wilson, Edward R. Winga,
> Joseph W. Edgett, and Thomas T. Gushiken,
> on behalf of the Executive Board, La Crosse
> Cardiac Rehabilitation Program.

Contents

PART I. POLICIES AND PROCEDURES

PART II: ILLUSTRATIVE MATERIALS

Contents

APPENDIX

part I

Policies and Procedures

chapter 1
Organizational Material

Organizational Material

I. HISTORICAL BACKGROUND

Based upon the premise that physical exercise would benefit patients with coronary heart disease (CHD), a discussion group was organized early in 1970 for the purpose of determining the feasibility of an exercise-oriented cardiac rehabilitation program for the La Crosse area. This group was comprised of representatives of the La Crosse area medical profession, the Wisconsin Heart Association, and the University of Wisconsin-La Crosse. During the month of October, 1970, representatives of the discussion group visited and observed cardiac rehabilitation programs at the following locations: Cleveland Jewish Community Center; Bio-dynamics Laboratory of the University of Wisconsin-Madison; University of San Francisco; and San Diego State University. Much of the foundation of the La Crosse Cardiac Rehabilitation Program was built upon aspects of these four programs.

In April, 1971, an Executive Board was established for the La Crosse Cardiac Rehabilitation Program, with the Wisconsin Heart Association, one lay individual, the medical clinics and hospitals of the City of La

Crosse, and the University of Wisconsin-La Crosse represented in its membership. Positions established on the Executive Board were: Chairman, Associate Chairman, Secretary, and Program Director. The program was to be operated on an experimental basis for one year (June, 1971 to June, 1972). At the end of that time an evaluation took place to decide whether the program should continue.

The program was sponsored directly by the School of Health, Physical Education, and Recreation of the University of Wisconsin-La Crosse, with the cooperation of the Wisconsin Heart Association, the medical clinics and hospitals within the La Crosse area, and the La Crosse County Medical Society. Professional liability and malpractice insurance coverage was provided. The initial funding of the program came from the University of Wisconsin-La Crosse, Gundersen Clinic, Ltd., and the La Crosse County Medical Society. The participating patients paid a monthly fee of $25.00. Program brochures were sent to area physicians for use in explaining the program to potential participants. The program consisted of three exercise sessions per week and periodic laboratory evaluations. At the conclusion of the first year of operation, the "experimental year data" were examined and it was decided to offer the program on a permanent basis.

The rehabilitation program was expanded in November, 1972, with the establishment of an Advanced Exercise Group, composed of those patients who had progressed through three months of swimming pool exercise and three months of track exercise. The Advanced Group exercised twice weekly, and their exercise was not under the supervision of a physician.

II. OBJECTIVES.

The objectives of the La Crosse Cardiac Rehabilitation Program are as follows:

A. To provide an opportunity for cardiac patients (nonoperative and postoperative) and those considered prone to coronary heart disease to become involved in a scientifically and medically sound exercise program.

B. To provide guidance and supervision in the use of exercise as a form of therapy in the rehabilitation of patients with cardiac disease.

C. To periodically determine, through laboratory evaluation, the most advantageous exercise level for the program participants.

D. To educate the program participants in regard to the cardiovascular and related benefits available through controlled, progressive, physical exercise.

E. To provide physicians of the La Crosse area with an opportunity to refer cardiac patients and those considered prone to coronary heart disease to a quality exercise program, from which they would receive data pertinent to the patient's laboratory evaluation and monthly exercise progress.

chapter 2

Administrative Material

Administrative Material

I. EXECUTIVE BOARD

A. The Executive Board of the Cardiac Rehabilitation Program should be composed of representative members of the medical profession in the community and the affiliated academic community (e.g., the Department of Physical Education of a college or university that provides facilities and personnel for the program) and at least one lay person. The local chapter of the American Heart Association should also be represented on the board. The Program Director and the Associate Director are members of the board.

B. New members are selected by majority vote of present board members.

C. Board members participate on a volunteer basis.

D. A member may resign from the board or is automatically removed from the board upon poor attendance at board meetings.

E. Quarterly meetings are arranged by the Program Director.

F. Medical Director, Associate Medical Director, Program Director, and Associate Director are chosen for three-year terms by a majority vote of the Executive Board.

G. This board or the Medical Director may appoint members or nonmembers to appropriate committees.

H. Current Committees

    1. Program Evaluation Committee

    2. Budget and Finance Committee

    3. Research Committee

    4. Nominating Committee

I. The Program Director and Medical Director serve on all committees.

J. A monthly summary is sent to the Executive Board members by the Program Director (Figure 1).

II. PATIENT REFERRAL, ACCEPTANCE CRITERIA, PROGRAM ENTRANCE

A. Categories

Two categories of patients are accepted into the program after appropriate physician referral and approval of the referral by the Medical Director or Associate Medical Director (Figure 2):

1. Cardiac-Prone Patients

This includes persons with hyperlipidemia, hypertension, diabetes mellitus, and/or a strong family history of premature CHD.

2. Cardiac Patients

This includes patients with known coronary heart disease. The University Cardiac Rehabilitation Program is considered the third phase of rehabilitation for cardiac patients who have been referred. Ideally, the patient will have passed through Phase I of cardiac rehabilitation while in the hospital, and Phase II, at home (see Chapter 4).

B. Additional Qualifying Factors

1. The patient should be physically capable of performing exercise.

2. A physician referral form must be completed by the patient's personal physician prior to the initial laboratory evaluation (Figures 3 and 4).

3. The patient must not be in congestive heart failure.

4. Angina must have been stable for one month.

5. Two months must have elapsed from the time of infarction prior to entrance into the program.

6. Two months must have elapsed from the time of cardiac surgery prior to entrance into the program.

C. Contraindications

1. Cardiac-Prone Patients

   Those patients who are prone to CHD owing to various coronary artery disease minor risk factors (such as physically sedentary, obesity, type A personality, smoker) will not be accepted into the program.

2. Cardiac Patients

   Patients with obstructive valvular heart disease and marginal cardiac compensation will not be accepted into the program.

D. Scheduling

Upon expressing interest in the program and being referred and approved for acceptance in the program, the patient will be scheduled for a laboratory evaluation and will receive a "welcome letter" (Figure 5) with an explanation of the laboratory evaluation (Figure 6), fees, billing, insurance and attendance procedures (Figure 7).

E. Advanced Group

Upon completing three months in the swimming pool, being re-evaluated and completing three months in the track exercise group, the patient will be re-evaluated and considered for transfer to the Advanced Exercise Group (not supervised by a physician). If transfer is approved by the Medical Director or Associate Medical Director, the patient and the primary physician are contacted for permission to transfer.

F. Re-referral

1. If a patient develops a change in symptoms or a contraindication to continuation in the program during a laboratory evaluation, exercise session, or outside the facility, he will be re-referred to his primary physician. The primary physician will be notified by phone or by letter and will receive a re-referral form (Figure 8).

2. The Re-referral Form regarding the new status of the patient must be filled out by the primary physician before the patient can again participate in the Cardiac Rehabilitation Program.

G. Termination of Participation

The participant is required to attend 70 percent of the scheduled exercise sessions per month, other than absences due to medical reasons, extended travel, or approved business commitments. A monthly list of patients placed on probation will be maintained (Figure 9). Upon being placed on probation, the patient (Figure 10) and the primary physician (Figure 11) will be notified. If the attendance does not improve during the one month probationary period, the primary physician will be notified that the patient is being dropped from the program and the patient will receive a copy of the memo (Figure 12). If the attendance during the probationary month improves appropriately, the primary physician will be notified of the cancellation of the probationary status and the patient will receive a copy of the memo (Figure 13).

III. FINANCIAL CONSIDERATIONS

A. Patient Fees

1. Laboratory Evaluations

The fee for the laboratory evaluation procedures is flexible and consistent with related area medical fees (Figure 7).

2. Exercise Therapy Sessions

The patient fees for the exercise therapy sessions are flexible and may be readjusted when appropriate (Figure 7).

B. Billing Procedures

1. Laboratory Evaluations. Upon completion of scheduled laboratory evaluation procedures, the Laboratory Evaluation Check List is delivered to the program secretary (Figure 14). The patient is then billed for the amount due.

2. Exercise Therapy Sessions. The patient is billed monthly for exercise therapy session fees (Figure 15).

3. The bill must be signed by the Medical Director.

4. Upon receipt of the appropriate amount, the patient receives a copy of the bill marked "paid."

C. **Insurance Claims**

1. These procedures will be followed regarding insurance claims:

   a. The participant is billed directly for all services provided during a laboratory evaluation.
   b. The laboratory evaluation services are included in the bill that the participant receives for the exercise therapy sessions.
   c. The participant is required to immediately reimburse the program for services rendered and not to withhold payment pending action by his insurance company.
   d. Attempts to obtain insurance company coverage for laboratory evaluation and exercise therapy session fees are to be made by the participant to his insurance company.
   e. The Cardiac Rehabilitation Program will file all Blue Cross/ Blue Shield claims, but payment must initially be made by the participant to the program.
   f. For non-Blue Cross/Blue Shield claims, the Cardiac Rehabilitation Program will provide the participant with information necessary to make the claim.
   g. Insurance coverage for laboratory evaluation and exercise therapy session fees is not guaranteed and varies greatly from company to company and within each company, depending upon individual insurance plans.

2. The patient is required to complete an Insurance Inquiry Sheet (Figure 16).

3. The patient is refunded or the account credited upon receipt of funds from third-party carriers. The patient is notified of such action.

D. **Assistance Fund**

An Assistance Fund is provided for those who cannot financially afford the established patient fees (Figure 17).

1. Authorization is by action of the Executive Board.

2. These applications are reviewed at the quarterly Executive Board meetings.

E. Delinquent Fees

The Program and/or Associate Director are to pursue delinquent fees. A series of four letters may be sent to the patient (Figures 18, 19, 20, 21). Failure to pay the requested amount upon receipt of the fourth letter entails automatic termination of program participation for active members.

F. Grants and Donations

The Program Director and appropriately designated individuals are permitted to apply for grants and/or donations to the Cardiac Rehabilitation Program from individuals, institutions, agencies or foundations.

G. Salaries

1. The Program Director and the Associate Director shall receive an annual salary for services rendered.

2. Graduate Assistants, Program Assistants, and Postdoctoral Research Fellows will receive a yearly salary decided upon by the Board.

3. Secretaries and other civil service personnel will receive the appropriate salary and fringe benefits as per their classification.

4. All salaries are subject to change on an annual basis upon decision of a majority of the Executive Board.

IV. SCHEDULING

The initial laboratory evaluation and all periodic laboratory evaluations must be scheduled by the Program or Associate Director. A Laboratory Evaluation Flow Chart (Figure 22) and Monthly Laboratory Evaluation Schedule must be maintained (Figure 23).

chapter 3
Staff

chapter 3
Staff

I. STAFF POSITIONS

Under the program directorship are a number of staff positions (Figure 24). These staff members are responsible to the Program Director, who in turn is responsible to the Associate Medical Director and the Medical Director. Ultimate responsibility for the program rests with the Executive Board.

II. STAFF SELECTION PROCESS

Staff selection is based upon need, interest, and qualifications.

III. STAFF RESPONSIBILITIES

A. Direct Staff

The direct staff has specific and assigned responsibilities:

1. Head Laboratory Technician (Figure 25)

2. Assistant Laboratory Technician (Figure 26)

3. Program Assistant, Pool (Figure 27)

4. Exercise Leader, Pool (Figure 28)

5. Program Assistant, Track—Exercise (Figure 29)

6. Exercise Leader, Track—Exercise (Figure 30)

7. Program Assistant, Track—Patient Education (Figure 31)

8. Exercise Leader, Track—Patient Education (Figure 32)

B. Indirect Staff

1. Internships and Postdoctoral Fellowships

   The Cardiac Rehabilitation Program cooperates with area medical clinics and hospitals in placing and training exercise technicians and exercise leaders (M.S.-degree recipients) and providing experiences for postdoctoral fellowship personnel (Figure 33).

2. Attending Physicians and Supporting Paramedical Personnel

   a. Attending Physicians for the program are accepted on the basis of interest.
   b. No financial reimbursement is provided to an Attending Physician for services rendered.
   c. All Attending Physicians and supporting paramedical personnel (nutritionists, medical technologists, physical therapists) are appointed to university faculty status by the Chancellor.
   d. All Attending Physicians must receive an orientation session from a veteran Attending Physician prior to attending an exercise session or laboratory evaluation as the responsible physician.
   e. The Attending Physician has specific responsibilities (Figure 34).
   f. A four-month schedule is sent to the physicians by the Program Director or Associate Director one month prior to the effective date of the schedule; upon finalization, the scheduled physician must be available for the laboratory evaluation or exercise session or find a suitable replacement (Figures 35, 36).

3. Volunteers

   a. Volunteers are important in the daily work schedule of the Cardiac Rehabilitation Program.
   b. Volunteers usually participate for the following reasons:
      (1) class requirement (high school and college).
      (2) enjoyment and fun.
      (3) need to contribute.
   c. The volunteer manual explains the responsibilities of the volunteer (Figure 37).

Phase I and II Materials

Phase I and II Materials

I. INTRODUCTION

Cardiac rehabilitation ideally consists of three phases, from hospitalization through home care to a long-term maintenance program.

II. DESCRIPTION OF PROGRAM PHASES

A. Phase I, In-Hospital

1. Coronary care unit, 1 to 3 days (Figure 38).

2. Ward rehabilitation program, 4 to 14 days (Figure 39).

B. Phase II, Home Rehabilitation Program, 14 days to 2 months

Toward the conclusion of Phase I, the patient is presented with a *Cardiac Rehabilitation Home Program Manual* (Figure 40). The manual details various aspects of Phase II of the rehabilitation program (diet, do's and don'ts, symptoms, etc.), with specific reference to the Phase II Home Exercise Program.

C. **Phase III, Aggressive Maintenance Rehabilitation Phase, 2 to 12 months**

    1. Beginning phase, 1 to 6 months

    2. Advanced phase, 6 to 12 months

Graded Exercise Testing

chapter 5
Graded Exercise Testing

I. TESTING PARAMETERS

A. Introduction

Patients in the Beginning Group of a Phase III program receive a laboratory evaluation at three-month intervals. Upon being transferred to the Advanced Group of Phase III, patients receive a laboratory evaluation six and twelve months later, and on an annual basis thereafter.

B. Forms

The following forms are utilized throughout the Grade Exercise Test (GXT) sessions;

1. Medical history form, filled out by patient (Figure 41).

2. Liability release, signed by patient, physician, Program Director, and witness (Figure 42).

3. Pre-GXT data form (Figure 43).

4. Graded Exercise Test form (Figure 44).

5. Dietary information form, to be reviewed by the program nutritionist (Figure 45).

6. Consent form to take and use pictures (Figure 46).

II. PROCEDURES OF TESTING

A. Purpose and Objectives

A Graded Exercise Test may be administered for many reasons.
Figure 47 lists the various purposes of a Graded Exercise Test.

B. Phase I, II, III GXT Specifics

On a routine basis, the patient will be administered specific Graded
Exercise Tests in the various phases of cardiac rehabilitation (a
standard GXT Summary Form, Figure 49, may be utilized for all
types of Graded Exercise Tests):

1. Phase I

   Prior to discharge from the hospital, the post-myocardial infarction and postsurgical patient will receive a low-level Functional
   Graded Exercise Test (FGXT) (normally termination heart rate of
   130 or less), for the purpose of determining the presence of
   arrhythmias or significant ischemia with or without angina. If not
   contraindicated, an exercise prescription for involvement in the
   Phase II program will be written, based upon data from the
   discharge FGXT.

2. Phase II

   At the completion of Phase II (six to ten weeks following
   discharge), the patient will receive a symptom-limited maximal
   FGXT for the purpose of defining contraindications to continuation in the rehabilitation program and involvement in Phase III.

3. Phase III

   The Graded Exercise Test is conducted within the Phase III
   program to detect contraindications to exercise involvement and
   to gather data necessary to write or rewrite exercise prescriptions. The following procedures apply to all Functional Graded
   Exercise Tests conducted in the Phase III program.

a. FGXT termination or "cut-off" heart rate
  (1) The *Cooper's Heart Rate Prediction Table* will be utilized
      to determine the FGXT termination or cut-off heart rate
      (Figure 48).
  (2) The *FGXT* will be to a percentage of the individual's
      maximal heart rate determined from the prediction table
      (Figure 48). The specific percentages are determined by the
      status of patients in the Phase III program and their medical
      conditions (Figure 50).
  (3) *Exceptions*
      The following exceptions require modification of the per-
      centage and termination heart rate procedures.

      (a) The FGXT termination heart rate serves only as a
          guideline; it should be ignored in the presence of
          contraindications (e.g., unaccustomed symptoms, ECG
          abnormalities, fatigue).
      (b) A patient taking a beta-blocking drug (propranolol—
          Inderal) may be exercising at an energy cost level that is
          20 to 30 percent beyond the indicated heart rate. It may
          therefore be necessary to terminate the FGXT prior to
          attaining the cut-off heart rate without the presence of
          contraindicating symptoms other than fatigue.
      (c) In establishing the cut-off heart rate for a cardiac
          patient who is beyond the age of 45 and reviewing his
          first (65%, category poor) or second (75%, category
          good) FGXT, it may be necessary to exceed the estab-
          lished percentages and categories owing to an espe-
          cially low cut-off heart rate. Exceeding the established
          percentages and category must be done only with the
          knowledge and permission of the Medical Director. In
          no case may the FGXT cut-off heart rate exceed 85% of
          a patient's predicted maximal heart rate within the
          "good" category.
b. Frequency of the FGXT
  (1) For participants in the Beginning Exercise group (M-W-F,
      physician-supervised)

Evaluation No.	Months in Program	Exercise Area
1	0	Pool
2	3	Track
3	6 (and every three months thereafter)	Track

  (2) For participants in the Advanced Exercise Group (T-Th,
      nonphysician-supervised)

Evaluation No.		*Months in Program*	
As Advanced Participant	Accumulative	As Advanced Participant	Accumulative
1	4	0	6 months
2	5	6	12 months
3	6	12 (and every 12 months thereafter)	24 months

c. FGXT Protocol

Two standard FGXT protocols are utilized for all participants in the Phase III program (Figure 51). The Advanced Protocol (A-FGXT) is used only with the subsequent test of patients who have completed the beginning test protocol (B-FGXT) prior to attaining the established heart rate termination point.

d. ECG-GXT Recording Procedure

A standard 12-lead ECG-GXT recording procedure will be used for all Functional Graded Exercise Tests (Figure 52).

III. EXERCISE PRESCRIPTION

An exercise prescription must be developed for all participants in an exercise program.

A. Rules for Exercise Prescriptions

1. The exercise prescription must be developed from data collected during a Graded Exercise Test.

2. The developed exercise prescription must be significantly below (minimum, 10 b/min below) the point at which symptoms appear during the GXT (e.g., unaccustomed anginal pattern, arrhythmia, ECG changes, fatigue), or if the GXT was symptom free, the point of termination of the GXT.

3. The exercise session intensity of the patient must always be at or below the exercise prescription "target heart rate." The patient is required to repeatedly take his heart rate before, during, and after exercise to guarantee a heart rate at or below the exercise prescription "target heart rate."

B. Symptom Recognition

The patient and exercise leader must understand the implications of symptoms before, during, and between exercise sessions. Communication between the patient and the exercise leader regarding a change in symptoms must exist because of implications regarding the exercise prescription and possible re-referral of the patient to the primary physician.

C. Development Procedures

The prescriptive process will vary slightly depending upon whether the GXT is conducted in the Phase III exercise testing facility or another (referral) exercise testing facility.

1. GXT, Phase III Facility

   If the GXT is conducted in the Phase III facility, the following procedures must be followed:

   a. Initial Exercise Prescription

   (1) *Cardiac Patient.*

   With the exception of unusual cases (i.e., patients who are taking Inderal, those who have an arrhythmia, or a highly conditioned patient), the initial exercise prescription should be for a target heart rate of 20 b/10 sec. Therefore, the patient must receive a FGXT to a minimal rate of 130 b/min (21 to 23 b/10 sec) or greater. Upon actual participation of the patient in exercise, it may be necessary to vary the individual's exercise prescription downward because of failure to meet the recommended value. Under no circumstances may the exercise prescription (target heart rate) be varied upward beyond the limit of 10 b/min below the most recent FGXT termination point.

   (2) *Cardiac-Prone Patient.*

   The cardiac-prone patient will most often receive an initial exercise prescription between 22 and 23 b/10 sec, depending upon his physical condition and results from the FGXT. Again, the initial exercise prescription may not exceed the point of 10 b/min below the termination point of the most recent GXT. The exercise prescription may also have to be adjusted upon actual involvement of the patient in the exercise sessions.

   b. Subsequent Exercise Prescriptions

   For both the cardiac-prone and the cardiac patient, the exercise prescription will be increased with each subsequent evaluation until the physiologic status of maintenance is attained (normally six to twelve months of exercise involvement.) All subsequent exercise prescriptions from the initial exercise prescription must be based upon a repeat FGXT and patient interview. The appropriateness of the previous exercise prescription must be determined. If the patient has had difficulty attaining the previous prescription, it is unwise to establish a new and higher exercise prescription that will be even more difficult to attain. In contrast, if the previous exercise prescription was attained regularly, with no undue symptoms or excessive fatigue, and no contraindications arose from the repeat FGXT, a new and higher intensity exercise prescription would be appropriate.

2. FGXT From Other Than Phase III Facility.
If the FGXT is conducted within a cooperating facility, it is inappropriate to repeat the GXT provided that the patient's cardiac status (symptoms, etc.) has not changed, and the referral FGXT was conducted within the preceding 45 days. The exercise prescription procedures then may be the same as for a patient who receives a laboratory evaluation within the program laboratory. However, a word of caution is necessary upon accepting Graded Exercise Test data taken from another facility. Often the data are relative to a maximal GXT and one cannot simply subtract 10 b/min from the cut-off heart rate value to develop an exercise prescription. The exercise prescription must be developed from the heart rate value at which the test would have been terminated had a functional GXT been conducted within the Phase III program laboratory. This procedure is necessary, or the exercise prescription will be exceedingly high.

3. Examples.
The following examples illustrate the calculation of FGXT termination heart rates and the development of exercise prescriptions for participants in Phase III of cardiac rehabilitation.

a. Cardiac patient, first evaluation, age 33
   (1) Category: poor
   (2) Maximal predicted heart rate: 187
   (3) 65 percent GXT cut-off heart rate: 121
   (4) Exercise prescription: 108 b/min = 18 b/10 sec
b. Cardiac patient, second evaluation, age 51
   (1) Category: fair
   (2) Maximal predicted heart rate: 179
   (3) 75 percent GXT cut-off heart rate: 134
   (4) Exercise prescription: 120 b/min = 20 b/10 sec
c. Cardiac patient, third evaluation, age 42
   (1) Category: good
   (2) Maximal predicted heart rate: 185
   (3) 85 percent GXT cut-off heart rate: 157
   (4) Exercise prescription: 144 b/min = 24 b/10 sec
d. Cardiac-prone patient, first evaluation, age 59
   (1) Category: poor
   (2) Maximal predicted heart rate: 159
   (3) 85 percent GXT cut-off heart rate: 135
   (4) Exercise prescription: 126 b/min = 21 b/10 sec

    e. Cardiac-prone patient, second evaluation, age 37
      (1) Catgeory: fair
      (2) Maximal predicted heart rate: 189
      (3) 85 percent GXT cut-off heart rate: 160
      (4) Exercise prescription: 150 b/min=25 b/10 sec
    f. Cardiac-prone patient, third evaluation, age 46
      (1) Category: good
      (2) Maximal predicted heart rate: 183
      (3) 85 percent GXT cut-off heart rate: 155
      (4) Exercise prescription: 144 b/min=24 b/10 sec

IV. PROCEDURES FOLLOWING GRADED EXERCISE TEST

All program participants and referring physicians must receive pertinent data regarding each laboratory evaluation. Information and related forms regarding procedures for such communication are listed below.

A. Reports to Personal Physician

  1. Explanatory memos

    a. Memo to physician upon administration of first laboratory evaluation (Figure 53).
    b. Memos to physician upon administration of subsequent laboratory evaluations (Figure 54)

  2. Laboratory evaluation flow sheet (Figure 55).

B. Reports to Patient

  1. Explanation of involved parameters on laboratory evaluation (e.g., heart rate, blood pressure, fat percentage, cholesterol, GXT) (Figure 56).

  2. Related memos and laboratory evaluation flow sheet (Figures 57, 58, 59).

Exercise Session Material

chapter 6

Exercise Session Material

I. EXERCISE SESSION MATERIAL

    A. An exercise prescription form is filled out by the assigned Laboratory Technician (Figure 60). The prescription is reviewed by the Program Director.

    B. Patient orientation forms are distributed to new patients who are entering the pool phase of the cardiac rehabilitation program (Figure 61).

    C. Patients who have been in the program for three months and are ready for the track phase of the cardiac rehabilitation process are given the patient orientation form on the track (Figure 62).

II. EXERCISE SESSION PROCEDURES

    A. Location

    All exercise sessions are conducted within a pre-established exercise facility.

28

B. Time

5:00 to 6:00, Tuesday and Thursday for the Advanced Group;
Monday, Wednesday and Friday for the Beginning Group.

C. Mode

Advanced Group, choice of swimming pool or track exercise
(swimming or jogging); the Beginning Group, months 1, 2, and 3
swimming pool exercise (walking, semisupport swimming, swimming), and months 4, 5, and 6, track exercise (walking, jogging).

D. Procedure

The patient dresses in the appropriate exercise apparel, reports to
the exercise area, and obtains the determined low heart rate. Upon
arrival of the assigned Attending Physician, the patients are led
through 10 to 15 minutes of warm-up exercise, for the purpose of
slowly increasing the heart rate to the exercise point and to avoid
muscle and joint soreness the following day. Upon completion of the
warm-up period, the patients partake in 30 to 35 minutes of vigorous
exercise at the prescribed heart rate. The cool-down phase lasts 10
to 15 minutes, and involves slow, relaxing exercise for the purpose
of slowly decreasing the heart rate to the desirable exit value. The
patient is allowed to leave the exercise area upon obtaining five
consecutive low heart rates. The entire exercise routine of the
patient is controlled by the patient's heart-rate response. A daily
Exercise Session Data Sheet (Figure 63), indicating the appropriate
heart rate for the patient throughout the one hour, is used by the
staff worker for each session. The Exercise Session Data Sheet is
also used by an assistant to record the patient's weight, exercise
tolerance, and exercise heart rate. All exercise sessions are supervised by the Program Director, assigned Graduate Assistant(s) and
Program Assistants.

E. Any patient who experiences difficulty during an exercise session is
required to report such to the student exercise assistant, and
appropriate action will be taken. If a patient experiences difficulty in
the evening or at other times when not participating in the program,
he should call his personal physician.

III. ADVANCED GROUP

Upon being in the program for six months, the patient may be
transferred to the non-physician-supervised Tuesday-Thursday Ad-

vanced Group, if approved by (1) the Medical Director, (2) the Program Director, (3) the patient's personal physician, and (4) the patient (Figures 64, 65, 66, 67). The patient may remain in the Tuesday-Thursday Advanced Group while space is available.

IV. PATIENT DETERIORATION

A. The patient's personal physician is notified of any temporary leave from the program and involved circumstances.

B. If the patient is removed from the program for cardiac reasons, return to the program must be approved by the personal physician, who completes a Re-referral Form and by the consulting cardiologist after a repeat laboratory evaluation (Figure 68).

C. Patient Hospitalization. The patient's personal physician and the Medical Director are notified.

V. EXERCISE REPORTS

It is imperative that the patient and primary physician receive monthly information on the exercise status of the patient. The Exercise Session Progress Reports contain information on the following: (1) weight, (2) exercise prescription, (3) exercise tolerance, and (4) attendance (Figure 69). The procedure and involved reports are as follows:

A. Reports to Patient (Figure 70)

Explanatory Memo and Exercise Session Progress Reports are sent monthly.

B. Reports to the Personal Physician

Exercise Session Progress Report and Explanatory Memo are sent monthly (Figure 71).

C. Subsequent Progress Reports

These are sent on a monthly basis to both the patient and the physician (Figure 72).

chapter 7

Cardiopulmonary Resuscitation (CPR) Materials

chapter *7*

Cardiopulmonary Resuscitation (CPR) Materials

I. CPR PROCEDURES

Cardiopulmonary resuscitation (CPR) procedures should be developed with the total program in mind. The following are primary CPR concerns for a cardiac rehabilitation exercise program: specific emergency procedures for employees (Figure 73); general protocol to be memorized (Figure 74); protocols for performing CPR at swimming pool (Figure 75), track (Figure 76), and locker room (Figure 77); sign in sheet for CPR responsibilities (Figure 78). Personnel responsible for performing CPR should be qualified by having attended at least the American Heart Association basic rescue course; mock practice sessions should be held monthly.

II. EQUIPMENT CHECKS

The following are standard procedures regarding all CPR equipment: equipment must be available, easily accessible, meet electrical codes, and checked on a regular basis (Figures 79, 80, 81, 82).

Patient Education
Materials

Patient Education Materials

I. GENERAL EDUCATION PROGRAM

The primary objective of the General Education Program is to educate and inform the public about this country's number one killer, heart disease. The General Education Program is divided into the following areas:

A. Patient Counseling and Education

All participants in the program are informed and counseled about specific topics. After the initial counseling and information sessions, these topics are reinforced during the first month that the participants are in the swimming pool phase, during all follow-up laboratory evaluations, and at the initial entry to the track phase and to the advanced group. The topics include:

1. The purpose of graded exercise testing

2. The benefits of exercise

3. An explanation of test results

4. An explanation of exercise prescription

5. Pulse monitoring

6. Symptoms (type and significance)

7. Introduction to exercise sessions

   a. Swimming pool (for those entering to use the swimming pool phase)
   b. Track (for those entering the track phase)
   c. Advanced (for those entering the advanced phase)

B. Monthly Lectures

The primary objective of the monthly lecture is to educate and inform the public on specific topics related to heart disease. Each month a different topic is presented. These lectures are free and open to the public. Monthly topics may include the following:

1. Coronary artery disease—will it kill you?

2. Basic anatomy of the heart

3. Exercise and your heart

4. Nutrition and holiday entertaining (Figure 83)

5. Smoking and its effects on the heart

6. Stress and its effects on the heart

7. Nutrition and fitness

8. Sex and the cardiac patient

9. Hypertension

10. Cardiopulmonary resuscitation

C. Mini-Education Program

The Cardiac Rehabilitation Program provides a six-month series of mini lectures on topics that might be of interest to participants and their families. The program is open to the public and is free of charge. Each lecture is approximately 15 minutes long and the program starts at 4:40 and ends at 4:55 on scheduled exercise dates. At the end of six months (January to June, and July to December), topics are repeated. Some topics span a number of sessions, depending on their magnitude. Participants in the program are encouraged to suggest topics of interest. The scheduled mini-education program includes the following topics:

1. Principles of stretching warm-ups

2. Specific stretching exercises for specific muscles

3. Biomechanics of running

4. Running in the heat

5. Running in the cold

6. Shin splints

7. Ankle sprains

8. Knee pains

9. Low back pains

10. Blisters

11. What is a MET? Why is it important?

12. What happens when I exercise?

13. Valsalva—why is it important to me?

14. Balancing calories with exercise

15. Exercise prescription

16. You and your posture

17. Selecting physical activities for the heart patient

D. Demonstrations, Talks, and Discussions

The need for public information about the prevention, maintenance and rehabilitation of heart disease is continuous. Because of this need, program personnel are often called upon to give demonstrations, talks, and discussions. The Cardiac Rehabilitation Program tries to provide personnel with expertise to deal with specific topics for specific groups.

E. Volunteer Education Program

It is important to permit volunteers in the program to learn more about coronary artery disease. With this in mind, volunteers are required to attend in-service education programs. The topics include:

1. An introduction to the rehabilitation program

2. The exercise prescription

3. Cardiopulmonary resuscitation

4. Symptomatology

F. CPR Classes

The Cardiac Rehabilitation Program provides American Heart Association certification and cardiopulmonary resuscitation courses to the spouses and families of patients. The courses are provided every other month. The student-teacher ratio is kept to a level of 10 to 1. Recording manikins are utilized in this course.

II. BEHAVIOR MODIFICATION PROGRAMS

These programs are available to participants in the Cardiac Rehabilitation Program as well as the general public. Three behavior modification programs are available, which include stress reduction, smoking termination, and weight control. A brief description of each program follows:

A. Stress Reduction

Held in February and October; seven sessions, 1½ hours each session. The stress reduction program employs various relaxation techniques, including aspects of standard autogenics training, respiration exercises for special accomplishments, role playing, and communication skills (Figure 84).

B. Smoking Termination Program

Held in January and September; four sessions, two hours each session. By means of informality, interaction, and introspection, the program examines the reasons why people smoke, the individual's potential for stopping smoking, the psychology and sociology of smoking, and techniques for stopping smoking (Figure 85).

C. Weight Control

Open only to Cardiac Rehabilitation Program participants, this program provides individualized nutrition guidance. The nutritionist interviews participants during the exercise sessions and during the laboratory evaluations. The primary concern is to aid the participant in attaining and maintaining his ideal weight, serum cholesterol, and triglyceride levels.

III. SKILL DEVELOPMENT PROGRAM

The skill development program is available to participants in the advanced phase of the Cardiac Rehabilitation Program. Emphasis is placed on the development of skills and attitudes toward recreational activities as a supplement to jogging. Participants are allowed to learn activities such as fly-casting, backpacking, canoeing, spin-casting, bicycling, tennis, cross-country skiing, badminton, bowling, table tennis, and golf (Figure 86).

IV. LEARNING CENTER

A Cardiac Learning Center has been established at our institution to provide patients with information on the various aspects of cardiovascular disease. This facility is available for patients and students. It is utilized especially for individualized and/or small group educational experiences, pretest and post-test counseling, behavior modification counseling, reading room, audiovisual programs, learning systems, and leisure time counseling.

Individual learning cubicles are available for those who are interested in using teaching machines. Programmed texts and audiovisual learning programs are available on a variety of subjects dealing with heart disease. A cardiac patient education series has also been developed and involves the dissemination of information that is especially important and specific for participants of the Cardiac Rehabilitation Program.

V. DISSEMINATION OF MATERIALS

Informing the public about available programs is often neglected. This can be handled by a variety of means, usually at a minimal cost. Various methods of disseminating materials are direct mailing, radio and television publicity, and the distribution of brochures.

part II
Illustrative Materials

Fig. 1. Cardiac Rehabilitation Program Monthly Summary

Grand Totals	Present Totals	Referrals*	Dropped**	Length in Program
Total involved since inception (June, 1971)	Enrolled—			0– 3 mos.
	M–W–F—			4– 6 mos.
	T–Th—			7–12 mos.
Referred—	Male—			13–24 mos.
Accepted—	Female—			25–36 mos.
Total GXT's—	Conducted GXT's—			
Total Exercise Hours—	Exercise Hours—			
	% of Attendance—			

PATIENT STATUS

	Cardiac Prone	Post-Infarct	Post-Operative	Rheumatic H.D.	ASHD Non-MI	Other
Total Patients						
Male Patients						

Figure 1   41

Female Patients

*Classification of Patients
1. Cardiac Prone
2. Post-Myocardial Infarction
3. Postoperative
4. Rheumatic Heart Disease
5. ASHD Non-Myocardial Infarction
6. Other

**Reasons for Dropping
1. Business conflict
2. Moved out of area
3. Dissatisfaction with progress
4. Re-referred to personal physician
5. Deceased
6. Loss of interest
7. Graduated
8. Medical reasons
9. Distance
10. Personal
11. Vacation
12. Nonattendance

PATIENT FLOW CHART

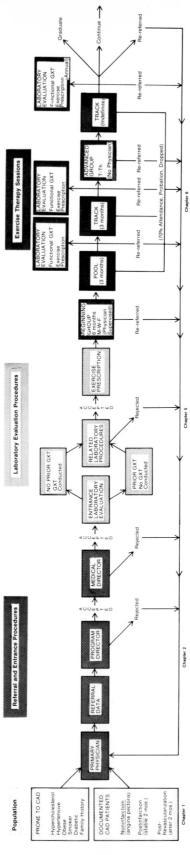

Fig. 2.

Figure 3   43

Fig. 3.   Physician Referral Form. Graded Exercise Test

Patient's Name ———————————————————— Date —————
Address ——————————————————— Age ——— Phone ———
    Street   City   State   Zip

Diagnostic Data

Etiologic	*Present Physical Activity*	*ECG*	*Rhythm*
1. No heart disease	1. Very active	1. Normal	1. Sinus
2. Rheumatic	2. Normal	2. Dig. effect only	2. Atrial fib.
3. Hypertension	3. Limited	3. Abnormal	3. Other
4. CAD	4. Very limited	4. Infarct	
5. Other			

Additional abnormalities you are aware of: ————————————
——————————————————————————————
Date of last complete physical examination: ————————————
Present medication: ————————————————————————
Please fill in the information below if it is available:
1. Urine, sp. gr. ——— Alb. ——— Glucose ——— Micro. ———
2. Complete blood count: Hbg. ——— Hct. ——— WBC ———
   Diff. ———
3. ECG, 12 lead (Enclose Copy) ——————————————————
4. Blood pressure, Syst. ——— Diast. ———
5. Cholesterol ——— mg.%   2 Hr. Post Dexicola ——— mg.%
6. Masters, and/or Graded Exercise Test Results (If available, enclose)

Impression of above information: ———————————————
——————————————————————————————

The above listed person is capable of participating in a Graded Exercise Test and related laboratory tests, conducted within the Cardiac Rehabilitation Program.

Signed: ———————————————————— (Physician)

Type or Print
Name of Physician ——————————————

Address ———————————————————— Telephone No. ———

Return to Program Director

Fig. 4.   Companion Memo to Physician Referral Form

TO: Primary Physician

FROM: Program Director
DATE:

    I have been contacted by _____, a patient of yours, relative to participation in the Cardiac Rehabilitation Program. Our program involves periodic laboratory evaluations and three exercise sessions per week for cardiac patients and those prone to coronary heart disease. All exercise sessions and laboratory evaluations are supervised by a physician. Enclosed is a brochure describing the program as well as a list of Attending Physicians for the program. Also enclosed is a referral form relative to _____which I would appreciate your completing and returning to me along with the patient's most recent electrocardiogram.

    Thank you for your cooperation. Please feel free to contact me if you have any questions concerning this matter.

    Return to Program Director.

Figure 5   45

Fig. 5. Welcome Letter

Dear _____:

    Welcome to the Cardiac Rehabilitation Program. We look forward to having you with us for your Laboratory Evaluation at (time) on (date) . You will begin the exercise phase of the program at (time) on (date) .

    Enclosed is an explanation of administrative aspects of the program as well as specific information regarding your upcoming Laboratory Evaluation. You will also find enclosed a list of the physicians who will be in attendance during our Laboratory Evaluations and Exercise Sessions. You will notice that we utilize physicians from all hospitals and clinics in the area.

    If you have any questions, please do not hesitate to call the Cardiac Rehabilitation Office. Again, welcome to the program.

Sincerely,

Program Director

Fig. 6.   Laboratory Evaluation Information

1. Name _____ Referring Physician _____
2. Your evaluation is scheduled at: _____, _____,
   _____.

3. Your Laboratory Evaluation will involve the following (items checked
   will be performed):
   _____ Interview, History, Risk Factor Examination
   _____ Anthropometric (Fat) Measurement
   Spirometry (Lung Measurements):
   _____   Vital Capacity
   _____   Forced Expiratory Volume (1 sec.)
   _____   Midexpiratory Flow Rate
   Electrocardiograms:
   _____   Supine
   _____   Standing
   _____   Posthyperventilation
   Blood Analysis:
   _____   Hemoglobin
   _____   Cholesterol
   _____   Hematocrit
   _____ Electrocardiographically monitored Graded Exercise Test
          (GXT) (Treadmill GXT, utilizing three-channel ECG recorder
          and three-channel companion oscilloscope and cardiotachome-
          ter, periodic heart rate and blood pressure determinations, and
          12-lead ECG recordings)
   _____ Nutrition Counseling
   _____ Exercise Prescription
4. Apparel (pertains only if you are scheduled for a Graded Exercise Test):
   Women—comfortable walking clothing and appropriate walking shoes
          as well as a button blouse with short sleeves that are very
          loose at the upper arm.
   Men—comfortable walking clothing and light walking shoes.
5. Please do not eat, drink, or smoke within three hours of reporting to the
   laboratory.
6. It is necessary that we record the names of all medications that you are
   currently taking. Please bring with you a bottle of each medication.
   The bottle may be empty, because we simply need to look at the
   prescription.
7. The physician in attendance for your evaluation will be _____
   _____ from _____.
8. Upon your arrival at the Human Performance Laboratory, please report
   to _____, ECG-GXT Head Technician.

Figure 6   47

9. If you are suffering from any temporary illness (such as cold, flu, or upset stomach), notify the Program Director so the scheduled test may be cancelled and a new appointment for the laboratory evaluation may be made.

10. If it looks as if you will be late, please notify the Program Director. If you have to cancel your appointment, let us know immediately because we would like to schedule another person in your spot.

Fig. 7.   Fees, Billing, Insurance, Attendance Procedures

The Cardiac Rehabilitation Program exists for the purpose of providing medically supervised Laboratory Evaluations and Exercise Therapy sessions for physician-referred individuals. The program is governed by an Executive Board that consists of representatives from area clinics and hospitals. Directly responsible to the Executive Board are a Program Director and Associate Director. The program is financed through fees charged to the participants for Laboratory Evaluation procedures and Exercise Therapy Sessions. Below is information regarding participant program involvement, fees, billing, insurance, and attendance procedures.

PARTICIPANT PROGRAM INVOLVEMENT

Each participant receives an Entrance (prepool) Laboratory Evaluation (LE 1) and is placed in the Beginning Exercise Group (exercise sessions Monday, Wednesday, Friday, 5:00-6:00 p.m.). A participant in the Beginning Exercise Group exercises in a swimming pool setting for three months, receives a second (pretrack) Laboratory Evaluation (LE 2), exercises in a track setting for three months, receives a third (pre-Advanced Exercise Group) Laboratory Evaluation (LE 3), and is then considered for transfer to the Advanced Exercise Group. Upon being transferred to the Advanced Exercise Group (exercise sessions Tuesday and Thursday, 4:30–6:00 p.m.), the individual receives a Laboratory Evaluation at twelve-month intervals. Below is a summary of the course of involvement of a participant in the program.

Beginning Exercise Therapy Group

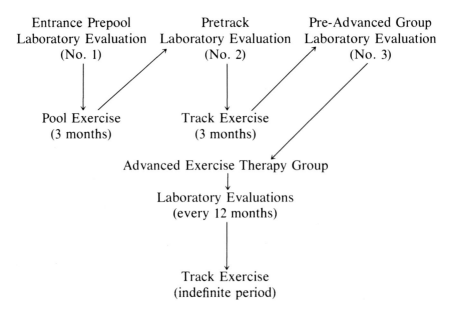

Entrance Prepool   Pretrack   Pre-Advanced Group
Laboratory Evaluation   Laboratory Evaluation   Laboratory Evaluation
        (No. 1)   (No. 2)   (No. 3)

Pool Exercise   Track Exercise
(3 months)   (3 months)

Advanced Exercise Therapy Group

Laboratory Evaluations
(every 12 months)

Track Exercise
(indefinite period)

Figure 7   49

Example:

Individual enters program .... January 1, 1976
Entrance prepool Laboratory Evaluation .... January 1, 1976
   (Pool exercise—3 months)
Pretrack Laboratory Evaluation .... April 1, 1976
   (Track exercise—3 months)
Pre-Advanced Group Laboratory Evaluation .... July 1, 1976
   (Enters Advanced Group—Track exercise
   for indefinite period)
Laboratory Evaluations (every 12 months)

A participant can enter the program at any time and is not required to make a commitment for a period beyond one month.

FEES

Below are the procedures conducted during the Laboratory Evaluations and the related fees (NC = no charge):

Interview, History, Risk Factor Examination .... NC

Anthropometric (Fat) Measurements .... NC

Electrocardiograms (ECG):
   Supine... $17.00
   Standing .... NC
   Posthyperventilation .... NC

Spirometry:
   Vital Capacity 5.00
   Forced Expiratory Volume (1 sec.) 5.00
   Midexpiratory Flow Rate 5.00

Blood Analysis:
   Cholesterol 6.50
   Hemoglobin .... NC
   Hematocrit... NC

Electrocardiographically Monitored Graded Exercise Test* 60.00
   (GXT). (Treadmill GXT, utilizing three-channel ECG
   recorder and three-channel companion oscilloscope and
   cardiotachometer, periodic HR and blood pressure
   determinations, and 12-lead ECG recordings.)

*A GXT conducted elsewhere within three months of referral from primary physician will be accepted, and entrance GXT within the Human Performance Laboratory will therefore not be conducted.

Exercise Prescription .... NC

Nutrition Counseling .... NC

TOTAL $98.50

Below are the fees for the *Exercise Therapy Sessions:*

Beginning Exercise Therapy Group .... $2.50 per session
                                     $30.00 per month (approximate)
    (M-W-F, 5:00–6:00 p.m., physician-supervised)

Advanced Exercise Therapy Group .... $2.00 per session
                                     $16.00 per month (approximate)
    (T-Th, 4:30–6:00 p.m., nonphysician supervised. Individual may come
    five times per week, but will be charged for two sessions per week.)

BILLING

At the beginning of the second month of participation in the program, each individual will receive a bill for all services rendered during the first month of participation. Each subsequent month, an itemized bill for the previous month will be mailed to the participant. Payment of the specified amount is expected promptly.

INSURANCE

The participant is *required* to pay the bill as soon as possible and *not* to withhold payment in anticipation of insurance coverage payment. The responsibility for the received bill rests with the participant. Attempts to obtain insurance coverage should be made by the participant to the individual's insurance company.

Many participants in the program will be able to obtain insurance coverage for Laboratory Evaluation fees and for Exercise Therapy Sessions; however, insurance coverage is not guaranteed. To assist in securing insurance benefits, the Cardiac Rehabilitation Office will provide each participant with a letter explaining the program, a program brochure, and a list of our Attending Physicians. This material should be sent with the bill (marked paid) to the participant's insurance company with a request for benefits.

With the exception of Blue Cross-Blue Shield, all insurance claims are to be filed by the participant to the company. If the necessary form requires the signature of a physician, the form should be submitted to the Rehabilitation Office. The form will be signed by the Medical Director and returned for the participant to complete and file with the insurance company. Blue Cross-

Figure 7   51

Blue Shield claims will be submitted by the Cardiac Rehabilitation Office, but again the payment must be made initially by the participant. The participant will be notified and receive a refund for all amounts received by the Rehabilitation Office for insurance claims.

ASSISTANCE FUND

An Assistance Fund has been created to financially aid those who would not otherwise be able to participate in the program. If a patient feels that utilization of funds through this source is necessary, an application form may be obtained from the Cardiac Rehabilitation Office. The application form will be considered by the Executive Board.

ATTENDANCE

A primary concern is that the individual attend the Exercise Therapy Sessions on a regular basis. It is illogical to expect benefits if the individual does not attend the Exercise Therapy Sessions regularly. The following procedures are to motivate the participant toward regular attendance:
1. The individual is billed for the number of sessions attended per month.
2. The participants and their physicians will receive a Monthly Progress Report. This report includes: (a) weight control, (b) prescribed heart rate, (c) exercise tolerance, and (d) attendance information. The attendance report will indicate "good attendance" if the individual attends a minimum of 90 percent of the sessions during the month, and "unsatisfactory attendance" if the attendance is below 70 percent.
3. If the attendance falls below 70 percent, the participant will be placed on probation. If the attendance rate does not reach 70 percent or greater during the following month the individual will be automatically dropped from the program. The individual's physician will receive written notification of probational status and, if necessary, removal from the program if satisfactory attendance does not occur during the probation period.
4. The individual is required to indicate either by telephone or previous message sessions that will not be attended. Sessions that are not attended are considered as absences.

EXCUSED ABSENCE

If the individual must miss a single Exercise Therapy Session for a valid reason (illness, business reasons, personal travel), the absence must be reported *before* the session that will be missed.

LEAVE OF ABSENCE

Individuals who must miss more than four weeks of Exercise Therapy Sessions will be considered to be on a leave of absence, and notification to

Theodore Lownik Library
Illinois Benedictine College
Lisle, Illinois 60532

the Cardiac Rehabilitation Office is required *before* the leave of absence. The following procedures will be in effect regarding a leave of absence:

Nonmedical Leave of Absence

a. *Less than 4 weeks.* Prior to resuming participation, the individual must be interviewed by the Program Director or Associate Director.

b. *4 to 8 weeks.* An interview is again required, and it may be necessary for the individual to receive a re-entry Laboratory Evaluation. Individuals in the Advanced Exercise Therapy Group will be required to exercise in the physician-supervised Beginning Exercise Therapy Group for one month prior to being returned to the Advanced Exercise Therapy Group.

c. *8 weeks or greater.* The participant's physician will be notified of re-entry into the program, and a Laboratory Evaluation will be required. Participants from the Advanced Exercise Therapy Group will be required to participate in the Beginning Exercise Therapy Group for one to two months prior to being returned to the Advanced Exercise Therapy Group.

Medical Leave of Absence

If a participant must take a leave of absence for medical reasons, the individual may return to the program after written permission from the primary physician is obtained by the Cardiac Rehabilitation Office. A re-entry Laboratory Evaluation may be necessary. Individuals from the Advanced Exercise Therapy Group may return to that group upon permission from the primary physician and after spending a period of time in the Beginning Exercise Therapy Group.

If you have any questions regarding this information, please feel free to contact the Cardiac Rehabilitation Office.

Figure 8   53

Fig. 8.   Re-referral Form

Patient's Name _____ Date _____
                      Last   First   Initial

Address _____ Telephone No. _____
              Street   City   State   Zip

Date of conducted laboratory evaluation or exercise session episode _____

YOU RECOMMEND:

_____ 1. Discontinue participation in the Cardiac Rehabilitation Program.

_____ 2. Temporarily discontinue participation in the Cardiac Rehabilitation Program while further investigation procedures be
conducted. Probable date of renewed participation. _____

_____ 3. Continue participation in the Cardiac Rehabilitation Program
while further investigative procedures be conducted. Probable
date of completion of investigative procedures _____

_____ 4. Continue participation in the Cardiac Rehabilitation Program. No
further investigative procedures to be conducted.

Physician's Name _____ Date _____

Physician's Signature _____

Summary of episode causing re-referral to primary physician:

Fig. 9.   Attendance Probation List (X For Probationary Month)

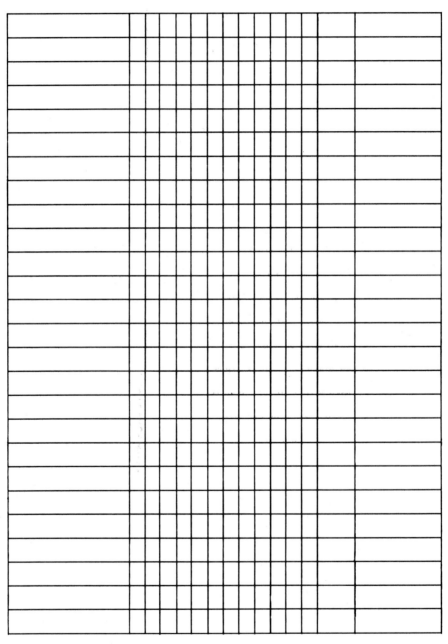

Figure 10   55

Fig. 10.   Probationary Notification—Patient

TO: Patient
FROM: Program Director
RE: Exercise Therapy Session Attendance

In checking our records, I find that your attendance at the Exercise Therapy Sessions for the month(s) indicated below has been very poor:

Month	Number of Sessions Attended	% of Total Sessions for the Month

If you are to be a participant in the program, it is very important that you attend a minimum of 70 percent of the sessions offered for that month. Since the attendance record shown above is far below 70 percent, you are being placed on PROBATION for the month of _____. If your attendance does not improve significantly during the probationary month, you will automatically be removed from the program.

　　If there are circumstances that justify your recent poor attendance, please contact the Cardiac Rehabilitation Office as soon as possible.

cc: Primary Physician

Fig. 11.   Probationary Notification—Physician

TO: Primary Physician
FROM: Program Director
RE: Patient Probation

    Enclosed you will find a carbon copy of a letter sent to ___(name)___ regarding his or her being placed on probation with the Cardiac Rehabilitation Program because of poor attendance.
    At the conclusion of the probationary period, ___(date)___, you will be notified of the status of the patient concerning continued participation in the program.
    Please feel free to contact me if you have any questions on this matter.

cc: Probationary Letter sent to patient

Figure 12   57

Fig. 12.   Termination Memo—Physician

TO: Primary Physician
FROM: Program Director
RE: Termination of Participation

    As you recall, _____, a patient of yours, has been a participant in the Cardiac Rehabilitation Program and was recently placed on probation because of poor attendance. The probationary period was from _____ to _____. During that time the patient has not shown an improvement in attendance. As previously stipulated, the patient is therefore being dropped from the rolls of the Cardiac Rehabilitation Program.

    If the patient again becomes interested in the program, I will contact you prior to his or her renewed participation. Please feel free to contact me if the patient does express such an interest to you.

    Please feel free to contact me if you have any questions. Thank you for your continued cooperation.

cc: Patient

Fig. 13.   Cancellation of Probationary Status

TO: Primary Physician
FROM: Program Director
RE: Termination of Probation Period

As you recall, _____ , a patient of yours, has been a participant in the Cardiac Rehabilitation Program and was recently placed on probation because of poor attendance. The probationary period was from _____ to _____. The patient has improved attendance during the probationary period and is to be removed from probation and will again be considered a fully instated participant in the program.

Please feel free to contact me if you have any questions. Thank you for your continued cooperation.

cc: Patient

Figure 14   59

Fig. 14.   Laboratory Evaluation Checklist

Patient _____
Laboratory Evaluation Date _____
            _____ Interview, History, Risk Factor Examination
            _____ Anthropometric Measurements

            Electrocardiograms:
_____   Supine
_____   Standing
_____   Posthyperventilation

            Spirometry:
_____   Vital Capacity
_____   Forced Expiratory Volume (1 sec.)
_____   Midexpiratory Flow Rate

            Blood Analysis:
_____   Cholesterol
_____   Hemoglobin
_____   Hematocrit
_____ Graded Exercise Test
_____ Exercise Prescription
_____ Nutrition Counseling

Comments:

Initialed by _____

Fig. 15.   Bill Format

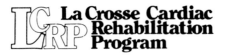

La Crosse Cardiac Rehabilitation Program

Mitchell Hall
University of Wisconsin-La Crosse
La Crosse, Wisconsin 54601
608/784-6050, Ext. 450
Joseph W. Edgett, M.D., Medical Director

DATE	DESCRIPTION	CHARGE	PAYMENT	BALANCE
	Balance Forward			

Please Pay This Amount ⟶

Referring Physician (Clinic) _____ Referral Date _____

Diagnosis _____

ECG	Electrocardiogram: 12-Lead Resting (93000)	ETX	Exercise Therapy Session (97100)
EST	Standing (93000)	IHR	Interview, History, Risk Factor Exam
EPH	Post Hyperventilation (93000)	APM	Anthropometric (FAT) Measurement
SVC	Spirometry: Vital Capacity (94150)	XRS	Exercise Prescription
SFE	FEV, 1.0 sec. (94160)	RFM	Risk Factor Modification Clinic
SMF	Mid Flow (94210)	UNF	Uniform
CHO	Blood Analysis: Cholesterol (82465)	ADJ	Adjustment
HGL	Hemoglobin (85050)	ASF	Assistance Fund
HCT	Hematocrit (85055)	INS	Insurance Payment
GXT	Graded Exercise Test (93260)	RFD	Refund

Joseph W. Edgett, M.D.   DATE
Medical Director, LCRP

Figure 16   61

Fig. 16.   Insurance Inquiry Sheet

Name _____ Birth Date _____

Address _____ Phone No. _____

_____

Physician _____

Address or Clinic _____

Insurance Company _____

Policy No. _____ Group No. _____

Address _____

Type of Insurance _____

Employer _____

Fig. 17.   Assistance Fund Application

Name _____ Date __/__/__
                 Last   First   Initial

Address _____
              Street   City   State   Zip

Age _____   Birth Date __/__/__   Home Phone _____

Marital Status: S M D W   Number & Ages of Children _____

Occupation (Present or Most Recent) _____

Employment Status (Please Circle): (1) Full Time (2) Part Time (hours per

week) _____ (3) Unemployed—Medical Reasons (4) Unemployed—Other

(5) Retired (If retired, how much are you receiving from pension or

retirement funds?) _____.

Employer _____Business Phone _____

Address _____

Monthly Salary _____

Other Income _____ Source _____

Spouse's Employer _____

Address _____

Monthly Salary _____

Bank _____ Checking _____

                                   Loan _____

                                   Savings _____

Do you have insurance coverage for: Exercise Sessions ____

                                      Lab Evaluations _____

Expenses and other financial circumstances that create this need (write on

back of sheet if needed) _____

_____

Figure 17   63

Please indicate how much you can afford to pay of the program costs:

Exercise Sessions are approximately $30.00 (Beginning Group) or $18.00 (Advanced Group) per month. I can afford paying _____ per month. Laboratory Evaluations cost $98.50. I can afford to pay _____ of this amount.

Signature of Applicant: _____

Fig. 18.   Delinquent Fee Letter No. 1

Date:

Dear _____:

   In checking our records for the Cardiac Rehabilitation Program, we find that you have been billed for the past several months with no resulting payment. Your present balance is $ ____. In that the operation of our Cardiac Rehabilitation Program depends heavily on payment of amounts due from patients, the failure on your part to pay the billed amount is placing participation by others in jeopardy. Would you, therefore, compensate the program for the amount involved as soon as possible.

   As I am sure you realize, the requested amount should be sent in check form to the Business Office. Please feel free to contact me if you have any questions on this matter.

Sincerely,

Program Director

Figure 19   65

Fig. 19.   Delinquent Fee Letter No. 2

Date

Dear _____:

   I am writing concerning the $_____ for the following periods of your participation in the Cardiac Rehabilitation Program:
   You received a letter on _/_/_ requesting payment of this amount, and at that time the bill was overdue for several months. The bill, therefore, is presently overdue for a period of _____. Your payment of the amount requested is of considerable concern to those of us who operate the Cardiac Rehabilitation Program, because failure on your part to pay the billed amount is placing participation by others in jeopardy. Therefore, if payment is not made within a reasonable period of time, appropriate action will be taken.
   I am sure you realize the requested amount should be sent in check form to the Business Office. Please feel free to contact me if you have any questions concerning this matter.

Sincerely,

Program Director

Fig. 20.   Delinquent Fee Letter No. 3

Date

Dear _____:

    I am writing to request payment for past due patient's fees you have incurred as a past participant in the Cardiac Rehabilitation Program. You are in debt to the program for the indicated amount for the periods indicated:

    You received a letter on _____, a second letter on _____ and were called on _____ concerning the amount owed to the program. Therefore, due to continued failure on your part to pay the requested amount, appropriate action will be taken if the amount is not received within 30 days.

    Please feel free to contact me if you have any questions concerning this matter.

Sincerely,

Program Director

Figure 21   67

Fig. 21.   Delinquent Fee Letter No. 4

Date

Dear _____:

    I am writing concerning the amount of money that you still owe the Cardiac Rehabilitation Program. You received letters requesting payment for the amount on the following dates:

    Below is an itemized statement of the amount owed:

    This is the fourth formal contact that I have been forced to make with you concerning the amount you owe, and therefore you should consider this the final contact. If payment is not received within 30 days, appropriate action will be taken.
    Please feel free to contact me if you have any question concerning this matter.

Sincerely,

Program Director

Cardiac Rehabilitation Program

Fig. 22.   Laboratory Evaluation Flow Chart

—Indicate months of lab evaluations

—M-W-F group   —T-Th group

Day	Name	Jan	Feb	Mar	Apr	May	Jun	Jul	Aug	Sept	Oct	Nov	Dec

Figure 23   69

Fig. 23.   Monthly Laboratory Evaluation Schedule

TIME	PATIENT	REFERRING PHYSICIAN	ATTENDING PHYSICIAN	DATE

Fig. 24. Staff Alignment

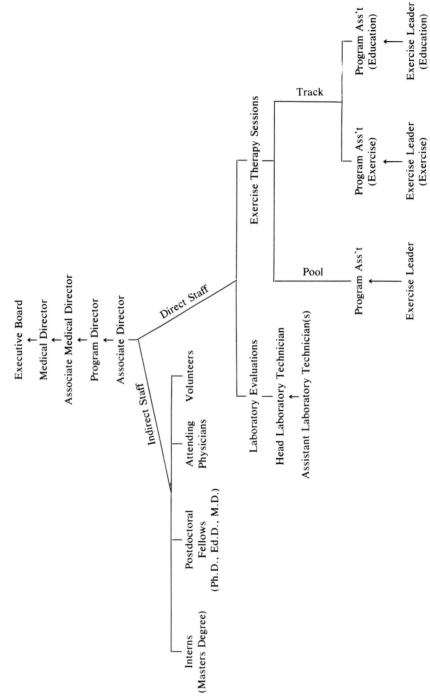

Figure 25   71

Fig. 25.   Head Laboratory Technician Responsibilities

1. The Head Laboratory Technician is responsible to the Program Director or Associate Director.
2. Present new patient cases to staff at weekly meetings.
3. Report at 2:00 p.m. to Human Performance Laboratory. Check defibrillator and sign defibrillator check sheet.
4. Check with Program Director's office for people to be evaluated (on clipboard).
5. Note who will have a GXT and who will have only a resting ECG.
6. Prepare appropriate forms for patients:
     A.   Informed consent
    *B.   Picture consent
    *C.   Medical history
     D.   Fat study
     E.   GXT test protocol
     F.   GXT comparative graph sheet
    *G.   Pool instructions
     H.   Track instructions (for those moving from pool)
     I.   Dietary information sheet
    *J.   Insurance and billing
    *K.   Exercise and caloric expenditure chart
    *L.   Book, *Exercise Your Heart* by Bill Maness (London, Collier Books, 1969.)
    *M.   Miscellaneous pamphlets
7. Fill out ECG data folder: Supine, Standing, Posthyperventilation, Name and Date.
8. Type labels for ECGs.
9. Check to see who is the physician for the day.
10. Assign patients to staff.
11. Determine appropriate GXT Termination Heart Rates.
12. Greet patients—introduce to staff and to student who will be doing the interview.
13. Oversee patient preparation and patient flow and assign duties to laboratory personnel.
14. Familiarize yourself with general patient histories, etc.
15. Greet physician, introduce him to patients, assistant laboratory technicians, and any visitors in the lab.
16. Oversee GXTs and organize patient flow for spirometric evaluation, blood analysis, and nutrition counseling.
17. Upon completion of GXT, prescribe exercise heart rates.

$$\text{Exercise HR} = \frac{\text{GXT Max. HR} - 10 \text{ beats per min.}}{6} = 10 \text{ sec H.R.}$$

*For new patients only

18. Fill out exercise prescription sheets; put one in folder and one to the pool or track recorder.
19. Patient Exit Interview
    A. Present data and test results to the patient.
       (1) Blood pressure—explain normal pattern during a GXT versus the patient's pattern.
       (2) Heart rate—explain normal relationship with exercise in comparison to the patient's recorded heart rate.
    B. Explain the exercise prescription.
       (1) What does it mean?
       (2) How do you use it in the track/pool?
       (3) When do you use it?
       (4) How can you use it in job-related physical activity?
    C. Demonstrate pulse monitoring
       (1) Demonstrate how to monitor the carotid pulse.
       (2) Practice trial—have patient take his HR (carotid pulse) while the lab technician checks him with a radial measurement.
    D. Introduce the patients to the Exercise Sessions by taking them verbally through a mock exercise session. Tell new patients about the pool, and others about the track. The following information must be covered:
       (1) Dress in locker room and weigh in before entering pool.
       (2) Take entering HR and report both weight and HR to person at desk.
       (3) Warm up exercises on land—random HR checks.
           Warm up exercises in the water—HR checks.
       (4) Exercise session begins: a. First two weeks, just walking with a pulse check every lap or two.
           b. Third or fourth week, begin to swim with a life belt (elementary backstroke).
           c. Reassure those who are poor swimmers or who can't swim that they will be helped individually.
           d. Progress to swimming laps and reporting your HR (must always remember to stay at or under your prescribed HR).
       (5) Cool down exercises in the water followed by five HR checks.
       (6) Report those five HR values to the recorder at the desk and go to shower.
       (7) Do not shower with cold or hot water, but use mild lukewarm water.
    E. Attendance Policies
       (1) Remind the patients how important it is for them not to miss the

Figure 25   73

exercise sessions. If they can't make it, they must call in and let us know why they aren't coming. Give them the phone number to call.

(2) Explain the probation policies that take effect after a patient has less than 70% attendance. Attendance the following month must be better or the patient will be dismissed from the program.

F. Billing and Fees. Bills for the exercise sessions will come monthly; payment should be made immediately.

G. Question and Answer period for patients to ask technician anything they fail to understand.

H. Reminder of where, when, and what to bring to the first exercise session.

(1) Time 4:45; date.

(2) Meet in Lab for the first day; otherwise, dress in the locker room.

(3) Bring a lock, towel, and bathing suit.

I. End with a word of encouragement ("Glad to have you with us. I'm sure you'll do just fine. See you in the pool.")

20. Summarize test results of all patients at weekly staff meetings.

21. See that lab is cleaned up and equipment is put away.

22. Throughout the lab evaluations, the Head Technician No. 1 will have two assistants: Assistant Technician No. 2 and Assistant Technician No. 3. The Head Technician No. 1 will utilize the two assistants in whatever way he or she feels will expedite the evaluations.

23. It is the Head Technician's responsibility to have the patients ready for the GXT prior to 4:00; thus, when the physician arrives, the GXTs can immediately start.

24. On Mondays, Wednesdays and Fridays when no lab evaluations are scheduled, the Head Technician helps with the track and swimming pool exercise sessions when needed.

Fig. 26. Assistant Laboratory Technician Responsibilities

1. Assistant Laboratory Technician is responsible to the Head Laboratory Technician.
2. Report at 2:00 to Human Performance Laboratory.
3. Set up prep tables:
    A. Alcohol swabs
    B. Razor and blades
    C. Towels
    D. Electrode cream
    E. Electrodes
    F. Sand paper
    G. Elastic bandage wraps (Ace)
    H. Cut tape
     I. Spray stick substances
    J. Electrode wires
    K. Preamplifiers
    L. Facial tissues
4. Check paper in ECG recorders.
5. Check preamplifiers and test electrodes.
6. Set up films—"Coronary Counter Attack" (for new patients); "Run Dick, Run Jane" (for follow-up GXT patients).
7. Learn assigned patient's history.
8. Set up chairs for viewers.
9. Set up blackboards, anthropometric instruments.
10. Patient Preparation Procedures:
    A. Interview, paying particular attention to present symptoms.
    B. Check patient's weight.
    C. Obtain signatures on all sheets calling for them.
    D. Take anthropometric measurements.
    E. Lay patient on table.
    F. Shave skin when and where necessary.
    G. Cream areas where electrodes are placed.
    H. Sand until skin is red.
     I. Swab with alcohol.
    J. Wipe with tissue.
    K. Take blood pressure.
    L. Apply electrodes; take supine ECG.
    M. Place recording in appropriate data folder.
    N. Tape electrodes.
    O. Stand patient up and wrap elastic bandage around leg leads and V leads.
    P. Take standing ECG.
    Q. Sit patient down on edge of table and have him hyperventilate for

Figure 26   75

20 seconds; keeping one hand on the patient's back. Take posthyperventilation ECG.
- R. Unplug electrodes.
- S. Send patient to spirometry station.
- T. Following spirometry, have patient fill out dietary information sheet.
- U. Show film to new patients.
- V. By 3:50, have two patients hooked up for GXT, seated on treadmills.
- W. Have appropriate information on the blackboards.
- X. Take pre-exercise ECG.
11. When physician arrives, explain patient's pertinent history to him and get his approval before administering GXT.
12. Warm patient up at 1.5 mph and 0% elevation for two minutes.
13. Sit patient down for two minutes.
14. Administer GXT:
- A. Take exercise ECGs every three minutes, using exercise set.
- B. Take full 12-lead ECGs for maximum exercise (Max. Ex.), immediate postexercise (I. P. E.), and recovery (2, 4, 6 min.).
15. Following GXT, direct assistants to remove electrodes.
16. Collect all ECGs and place them by folders.
17. Check with Head Technician No. 1 to see whether he or she needs help in counseling patients, prescribing heart rates, or filling out exercise prescription sheets.
18. Assist with clean-up:
- A. Clean electrodes.
- B. Makes sure preamplifiers are turned off.
- C. Replace ECG recorder.
- D. Rewind film.
- E. Take exercise prescription sheets to pool and/or track.
19. Assistant Technician No. 2 is second-in-charge, when the Head Technician is absent or has to leave. Assistant Technician No.3 is in charge when both the Head Technician and Assistant Technician No. 2 are absent.
20. On Mondays, Wednesdays, and Fridays when no lab evaluations are scheduled, assistant laboratory technician helps with the track and swimming pool exercise sessions when needed.

Fig. 27.   Program Assistant (Pool) Responsibilities

1. Program Assistant (Pool) is responsible to the Program Director or Associate Director.
2. Report no later than 4:55.
3. Oversee the entire pool phase of the Cardiac Rehabilitation Program. Be familiar with the responsibilities of the Exercise Leader (Pool).
4. Make sure assignments have been made for CPR. Test volunteers and Exercise Leader to assure yourself they know what to do in case of an emergency. If volunteers do not know what to do, seek out Exercise Leader (Pool) and make sure the necessary arrangements for proper protocol and coverage of CPR are made.
5. Know where the physician is at all times. Greet the physician when he arrives at the pool.
6. Orient new patients to the pool:
   A. Exercise procedure.
      (1) Weight check.
      (2) Entering heart rate.
      (3) Exercise procedure for first few weeks (check handout on Pool Phase of program, Figure 61).
   B. Swimming Procedure.
      (1) First two weeks—walking.
      (2) Elementary back stroke with life belt.
      (3) HR procedure after assigned laps.
   C. Cool-down procedure in the water.
      (1) Exercise.
      (2) Floating—one minute.
      (3) Obtain five ten-second HRs.
7. Follow-up on new patients in pool to be assured they are functioning well.
8. Answer questions on exercise for patients. Make yourself available to all patients.
9. General dissemination of information.
      Reinforce all information covered by Head Technician No. 1 during patient exit interviews (see Fig. 25, no. 19).
10. Each patient should be counseled daily in the pool. This means spending at least a few minutes at each session with *each patient* answering questions and reinforcing the patient's knowledge of what he is doing.

Figure 28   77

Fig. 28. Exercise Leader (Pool) Responsibilities

1. Present patients who have completed three (3) months in the pool and who are being evaluated to the staff at weekly staff meetings.
2. As Exercise Leader, you are directly responsible to the Program Assistant (Pool). Pool should be set up by 4:45. On the days on which lab evaluations are scheduled, report to the lab at 2:00 and help with the lab evaluations until 4:30. At 4:30, tell the Head Laboratory Technician that you are leaving to prepare the swimming pool for the afternoon session.
3. Pre-exercise responsibilities
    A. Set up equipment
        (1) Bring clipboard, heart rate and distance sheets, pencils, and student sign-in sheets to pool (4:45).
        (2) Unlock the doors.
        (3) Get out the following:
            a. Medications. (Contents and dates)
            b. Patient files.
            c. Tape player.
            d. Life belts.
        (4) Put out life-lines.
            a. Deep end.
            b. Walker's lanes.
        (5) Set up tables for patient's exercise sheets.
        (6) Set out the mats for exercises.
        (7) Get the music equipment ready.
    B. Go over emergency procedures with the student helpers (see Chapter 7). Make assignments.
    C. Assign student helpers to patients (walkers and new swimmers).
    D. Orient and introduce new patients. (If a Program Assistant is assigned, this will be his or her responsibility. However, during months when a Program Assistant is not assigned to the pool, it is your responsibility to orient the new patients.)
        (1) Exercise procedure.
            a. Weight check.
            b. Entering HR.
            c. Exercise procedure for first few weeks (check handout on Pool Phase of program, Figure 61).
        (2) Swimming procedure.
            a. First two weeks—walking.
            b. Elementary back stroke with life belt.
            c. HR procedure after assigned laps.
        (3) Cool-down procedure in the water.
            a. Exercises.
            b. Floating—one minute.
            c. Obtain five ten-second HRs.

E. Make sure the physician is in the building and make sure you know where he is before you start any exercises. Program Assistant should inform you when the physician has arrived and where he can be located.

4. Exercise responsibilities.
   A. Assign people to be lifeguards.
      (1) Helpers with individual patients.
      (2) Guards along the pool deck.
   B. Deck exercises (at beginning of month, introduce yourself and Program Assistant—Pool).
      (1) Series of five to eight different exercises. NO ISOMETRICS, NO BREATH-HOLDING, NO RIGOROUS STRETCHING EXERCISE, AND NO EXERCISES THAT ARE TAXING AND WILL RAPIDLY INCREASE THE HEART RATE.
      (2) One ten-second HR.
      (3) Continue with four to six more exercises.
      (4) One ten-second HR. Enter the shallow end of the pool, continue with warm-ups in the pool.
   C. Pool warm-up exercises (5 to 10 minutes). Stretch the shoulder girdle region and hip girdle region.
      (1) Exercises.
      (2) HR, and begin the swimming program.
   D. Safety
      (1) Constantly check to see whether the patients are feeling okay and progressing.
      (2). Make sure each patient is keeping his or her HR at a safe prescribed HR. Patients should be exercising at a rate of at least one to three heart beats below their prescribed maximum exercise heart rate. If a patient is over or at his prescribed HR, have him stop and rest for at least a minute or until his HR goes down to a safe rate.
      (3) Patient discomfort and pains. Be sure you understand the intensity of the pain. If you feel it is necessary, have the patient get out of the pool and call the physician. It's good idea to always record even the slightest pains. Never let a patient go down to the locker room without supervision. Make sure no patient leaves early without telling you why he or she is leaving.
   E. Pool cool-down procedure
      (1) Light exercises to relax and cool the patients down—five to ten minutes.
      (2) Supine floating—one minute. No movement.
      (3) Obtain five ten-second HRs.
      (4) Shower.
   F. Clean-up—the exact opposite of setting up the equipment.

Figure 29   79

Fig. 29. Program Assistant (Track, Exercise) Responsibilities

1. The Program Assistant (Track, Exercise) is responsible to the Program Director or Associate Director.
2. Report to track no later than 4:45. Check defibrillator and sign defibrillator check sheet. Prepare defibrillator and drug box in proper place.
3. Oversee the entire track phase of the program. Be familiar with the responsibilities of the Exercise Leader (Track, Exercise).
4. Make certain that assignments have been made for CPR. Test students and Exercise Leader to assure yourself that students know what to do in case of an emergency. If students or volunteers do not know what to do, seek out the Exercise Leader (Track, Exercise) and make certain that necessary arrangements for proper protocol and coverage of CPR are made.
5. You should know where the physician is at all times. Greet the physician when he arrives at the track. Inform the Exercise Leaders in charge of the pool and the track that the physician has arrived.
6. Orient new patients to the track. Be familiar with the handout on the Track Phase of the program (Figure 62). Go over the exercise procedures (duration and intensity) for the first few weeks.
7. Follow-up new patients in track to be certain that they are okay and functioning well.
8. Answer questions on exercise for patients. Make yourself available to all patients.
9. At 6:00 p.m., check defibrillator. Follow check-out protocol and sign check sheet.
10. Return defibrillator to battery charger.

Fig. 30. Exercise Leader (Track, Exercise) Responsibilities

1. Present patients who have completed three months in the track program and who are being evaluated to staff at weekly meetings.
2. As Exercise Leader (Track, Exercise), you are directly responsible to the Program Assistant (Track, Exercise). Track should be set up by 4:45. On days on which laboratory evaluations are scheduled, report to the lab at 2:00 and help with the lab evaluations until 4:30. At 4:30, tell Head Technician that you are leaving to prepare the track for the afternoon session.
3. Pre-exercise responsibilities.
   A. Set up equipment
      (1) Bring clipboard, heart rate and distance sheets, pencils and student sign-in sheets to track (4:45).
      (2) Make sure doors are unlocked.
      (3) Make sure defibrillator is plugged in and charged.
      (4) Get cabinets out and check the following:
          a. Patient files.
          b. Stereo-tape recorder.
      (5) Set up table for patients' exercise sheets.
   B. Go over emergency procedures (CPR) with student workers and volunteers. Make assignments. Check handout on CPR Protocol.
   C. Assign volunteers and regular employees to specific work responsibilities (setting up nets and equipment for skill development, recording heart rate and distances, running with participants, etc.).
   D. If no Program Assistant has been designated, orient and introduce new patients to track phase regarding the following:
      (1) Weight check.
      (2) Entering HR.
      (3) Go over exercise procedures for first few weeks (check handout on Track Phase of program, Figure 62).
   E. Make sure the physician is in the building and that you know where he is before you start any exercise. Program Assistant should inform you when the physician has arrived and where he can be located.
   F. Four times a month, set out the distance drum. (Drum containing total distance covered by participants.)
4. Exercise responsibilities.
   A. At beginning of month, introduce yourself, Program Assistant, and other workers.
   B. Warm-up exercises and heart rates:
      (1) Series of five to six different stretching and flexibility exercises. No holding of breath!
      (2) Obtain one ten-second heart rate.
      (3) Continue with four to six more exercises.
      (4) Obtain one ten-second heart rate, and start the walk-jog exercise.

Figure 30   81

C. The walk-jog exercise should be progressively increased over a period of two to three weeks.

D. Be available to answer questions on exercise and health.

E. Be pleasant, talk to everyone. Don't favor specific individuals. Constantly check to see whether patients are feeling okay and progressing.

F. Make sure patients are keeping their heart rates at a safe, prescribed level.

G. Patient discomfort and pains—be sure you understand symptoms. If a patient feels any discomfort, call the physician. Record and document all pains and symptoms. Never allow a patient to go to the locker rooms without supervision. Make sure no patient leaves early without telling you why he or she is leaving.

H. Make sure you know where the physician is at all times.

I. Supervise volunteers and other employees.

J. Track cool-down procedures.
   (1) Light stretching exercises for five to ten minutes on the track floor.
   (2) Obtain one ten-second HR.
   (3) Have patients lie down and breathe deeply for one minute.
   (4) Obtain one ten-second HR.
   (5) Shower.

K. Clean up—collect all paper work, make sure no one in the program is still running. Take paper work to lab, take down stereo, help put away equipment.

Fig. 31. Program Assistant (Track, Patient Education) Responsibilities

1. Program Assistant (Track, Patient Education) is responsible to the Program Director or Associate Director.
2. Report no later than 4:50 p.m.
3. When no Program Assistant (Track, Exercise) has been assigned for a particular month, you will assume those designated responsibilities.
4. Otherwise, the following are your responsibilities:
   A. Set up question and answer sign at an area close to the check-in tables.
   B. Work with Exercise Leader (Track, Patient Education).
      Know his or her responsibilities (Figure 32) and make sure they are being carried out.
   C. Assist in teaching the lifetime sports.
   D. Advise the Exercise Leader on how to organize and get people involved in the Skill Development Program.
   E. Reinforce all information covered by Head Technician No. 1 during patient exit interviews.
   F. Each new patient on the track should be counseled daily for the first month. This means spending at least a few minutes at each session answering questions and reinforcing the patient's knowledge about what he is doing.

Figure 32   83

Fig. 32.   Exercise Leader (Track, Patient Education) Responsibilities

1. As Exercise Leader (Track, Patient Education), you will be directly responsible to the Program Assistant who is in charge of Track, Patient Education.
2. Your responsibilities include:
   A. Setting up blood pressure screening.
   B. Skill Development
       (1) Set up equipment and nets for volleyball, golf, badminton and tennis no later than 5:00.
       (2) Secure student help or volunteers from Exercise Leader (Track, Exercise) to help set up and take down nets and equipment.
       (3) At 5:15, advanced patients can participate in the skill development program if they have completed their workout.
       (4) Beginning patients (nonadvanced) can participate in the skill development program at 5:35 or after they have completed their workout, whichever comes *later*.
       (5) Encourage all participants to become active in at least one lifetime activity.
       (6) Be familiar with the rules and skills of each activity. Be able to teach each activity if necessary. Patients understand that you are not a professional.
       (7) Make certain that patients take their pulse rates at regular intervals while participating in the Skill Development Program.
       (8) All of our skills should de-emphasize competition. We also need to emphasize these activities as supplements to the aggressive exercise program, *not* as alternatives.
   C. Public Relations—Patient Education Program.
       Develop patient interest in the Patient Education Program. One week before program, encourage participants to attend with their families and friends.
   D. General Dissemination of Information.
       (1) Reinforce all information covered by Head Technician No. 1 during patient exit interviews.
       (2) Each new patient in the track program should be counseled daily for the first month. This means spending at least a few minutes at each session answering questions and reinforcing the patient's knowledge of what he is doing.

Fig. 33.
Internships (M.S. Degree) and Postdoctoral Fellowships (M.D., PhD., Ed.D.)

The Policies and Procedures listed below have been developed to govern the Cardiac Rehabilitation Internship as a cooperative effort of area medical clinics and hospitals and the Cardiac Rehabilitation Program.

I.   RESPONSIBILITIES OF RECIPIENT: The internship is for a period of fifteen (15) months, specified as three (3) months of training, and twelve (12) months of clinic and laboratory experience.
   A. Training Period (Months 1, 2 and 3)
      1. Training within Human Performance Laboratory of the University involving:
         a. Successful completion of specified graduate courses.
         b. Demonstration of necessary statistical competencies or completion of appropriate graduate level course.
         c. Direct involvement in functional GXTs.
         d. Direct involvement in operational procedures of the University phase (Phase III) of the Cardiac Rehabilitation Program.
      2. Training within Exercise Laboratory of involved medical clinic/ hospital, and related areas, involving:
         a. Indoctrination of procedures through direct supervision by present Exercise Technician (final 3 months of internship).
         b. Involvement in in-service education programs resulting in overall concept of purposes of Graded Exercise Testing and related laboratory responsibilities.
         c. Awareness and understanding of Phases I and II of the Cardiac Rehabilitation Program.
         d. Successful completion of an instructor's level Cardiac Rehabilitation course.
   B. Clinic and Laboratory Experience (Months 4 through 15)
      1. Exercise Laboratory of medical clinic/hospital (10 a.m. to 3:00 p.m., M-F)
         a. Conduct, under direct supervision of appropriate physician(s), Graded Exercise Tests.
         b. Additional responsibilities as related to purpose of the laboratory.
      2. Human Performance Laboratory (9:00-10:00 a.m., 3:30-6:30 p.m., M-F)
         a. Operational and administrative responsibilities.
         b. Assist in conducting laboratory evaluations and exercise sessions.

Figure 33   85

3. Research responsibilities (in addition to foregoing specified time periods)
   a. Development of two (2) research projects relative to "Exercise and the Cardiovascular System."
   b. Presentation of research proposals to Research Committee (Subcommittee of Executive Board, Cardiac Rehabilitation Program).
   c. Conduction, completion and possible publication of approved research projects.

II. RESPONSIBILITIES OF INVOLVED MEDICAL CLINIC/HOSPITAL AND CARDIAC REHABILITATION PROGRAM

A. Cardiac Rehabilitation Program, University
   1. Place individuals who would be potential appointees and, with training, competent as an Exercise Technician.
   2. Provide an office and related study and research areas.
   3. Educate the selected individual in the physiologic concepts and laboratory techniques relative to Graded Exercise Testing and related parameters.
   4. Supervise the selected individual during involvement in laboratory evaluations, exercise sessions, and administrative aspects of the university phase of the rehabilitation program.
   5. Supervise and advise on research projects, as approved and directed by the Research Committee.
   6. Make available to the intern the use of Human Performance Laboratory, Computer Center, and additional university areas as necessary for research efforts.
   7. Additional supervisory and educational responsibilities of appointee, as determined by appropriate individuals.

B. Medical Clinic/Hospital
   1. Select individuals for internship, based upon information and recommendations of the Director of the Cardiac Rehabilitation Program.
   2. Employ the intern from the period of August 1 through July 31.
   3. Supervise and instruct the intern, as dictated by expected work responsibilities, beyond the scope of the training period learning experiences.
   4. Provide the opportunity for the intern to attend "in-service" education courses and lectures, if not in conflict with work responsibilities.

III. RESEARCH RESPONSIBILITIES (RESEARCH COMMITTEE, EXECUTIVE BOARD, CARDIAC REHABILITATION PROGRAM)

A. The Research Committee is responsible for advising and supervising the intern on research efforts through the involved agencies.
B. The intern will be expected to complete all research projects (including publication preparations if appropriate) and report upon such to the Research Committee prior to completion of the internship.

The foregoing policies and procedures may be modified at any time. However, the financial arrangements are binding for the yearly appointee to an internship position.

Figure 34   87

Fig. 34.   Attending Physician Responsibilities

I.   LABORATORY EVALUATION
   A. Pre-Graded Exercise Test Responsibilities
      1. Screen patient concerning the following:
         a. Drug usage
         b. Work tolerance
         c. Chest pain
      2. Observe ECGs and report irregularities to Program Director:
         a. Referral ECG
         b. Supine ECG
         c. Standing ECG
         d. Posthyperventilation ECG
      3. Study referral information and previous laboratory evaluation information on patient, relevant to contraindication for or manner in administration of the Graded Exercise Test (GXT).
      4. Examine emergency supplies and equipment.
      5. Decide whether the GXT is to be conducted.
   B. Graded Exercise Test (GXT) Responsibilities
      1. Communicate with Program Director concerning undesirable response of patient to exercise (GXT) in regard to following:
         a. Heart rate
         b. Blood pressure
         c. ECG
         d. Other
      2. Observe patient and communicate with the Program Director regarding undesirable visible patient signs of pallor, dyspnea, posture, etc.
      3. Query patient in regard to chest pain or other symptoms during exercise.
      4. Communicate with Program Director concerning cessation of GXT due to visible and/or physiologic signs indicating contraindication of further exercise.
      5. Be prepared to implement appropriate emergency procedures.
   C. Post-Graded Exercise Test Responsibilities
      1. Communicate with Program Director concerning irregularities in patient's recovery involving parameters of:
         a. Heart rate
         b. Blood Pressure
         c. ECG
      2. Observe and query patient about general feeling and sensations.
      3. Study exercise and recovery ECGs and make a decision concerning ST segment abnormalities.

4. Summarize in writing any unusual happenings or findings during entire laboratory evaluation. Summarization will be forwarded to the patient's primary physician.

II. EXERCISE SESSIONS

A. Report to exercise session by at least 4:55 p.m.
B. Notify Program Director or previously designated individual of your arrival.
C. Check the defibrillator to be sure it is in proper operating condition.
D. Check the drug box and oxygen tank.
E. You are encouraged to participate in the exercise (run or swim) sessions.
F. Someone will keep you in touch with the other exercise area.
G. If serious trouble should occur, students will aid in resuscitation and one will phone for an ambulance at your request.
H. If a patient is having symptoms of which the patient's primary physician is unaware or that preclude him from conducting his usual exercise (i.e., chest pain, increased shortness of breath, arrhythmia), he should be encouraged to recheck with his primary physician before re-entering the program. Give written summary of the incident to the Program Director or previously designated individual.

III. EMERGENCY PROCEDURES

A. Cardiopulmonary Resuscitation

1. *Open Airway*
Remove any foreign bodies; tilt head backward as much as possible and pull mandible forward.
2. *To Restore Breathing*
Plastic airway is available and one can give mouth-to-mouth respiration or use a ventilation bag with face mask and O_2 catheter. About 12 respirations per minute are generally adequate for ventilation.
3. *To Restore Circulation*
Initially, if no pulse can be detected, place patient on a firm surface, deliver a sharp blow to the sternum, and begin external cardiac compression over lower one-half of sternum at a rate of about 60/min.
Ventilate after every five compressions. Periodically check for the return of the carotid or femoral pulse. Check pupils periodically.
4. *Definitive Therapy* (Physician only)
Patient will be hooked up to ECG monitor.

Figure 34   89

a. Ventricular fibrillation—use defibrillator.

b. Cardiac standstill or straight line—may use 1 ml. epinephrine 1:1000 with 9 ml. of saline injected intracardiac or I.V.

c. I.V.: Put in when possible—a bottle of 500 ml. of D_5W with Saftiset is available.

d. NaHCO$_3$—May give one ampule (50 ml. or 44.3 mEq.) every 10 minutes.

e. Other drugs:

(1) Nitroglycerin—1/150

(2) Meperidine (Demerol)—75 mg.

(3) Epinephrine (Adrenalin)—1:1000—1 ml.

(4) Lanatoside (Cedilanid)—0.4 mg. in 2 ml.; 0.8 mg. in 4 ml.

(5) 1% Phenylephrine (Neo-Synephrine)—5 ml.

(6) Lidocaine—50 mg.

(7) Atropine sulfate—10 ml. of 0.4 mg./ml.

(8) Calcium chloride—10 ml.; 1 gm.

B. Defibrillation

1. *Large Machine* (permanent "plug-in")

a. Plug the cable of the paddles into "patient leads" (color-coded 3 yellow dots).

b. Cardioverter-defibrillator switches (color-coded 1 yellow dot) should be on "defibrillator."

c. Power switches on (color-coded 4 yellow dots).

d. Intensity dial (color-coded 5 yellow dots) turned clockwise until watt-second meter (color-coded also 5 yellow dots) reads 200 watt-seconds or more, as desired.

e. When meter shows capacitor is charged and paddles are in position on the patient's chest, press "manual discharge" (color-coded 6 yellow dots).

The upper three banks of controls regulate the ECG monitor and are not needed in defibrillation. Delay switch (color-coded 2 yellow dots) is for elective cardioversion and is not used in defibrillation.

2. *LifePak/33* (Battery-Operated DC Defibrillator)

a. Turn main power switch *ON*. Green light will be on if battery is functional.

b. Apply Derma-Jel to paddles.

c. Place paddles firmly on chest.

d. Observe oscilloscope and adjust *QRS height control* if necessary.

e. Rotate *watt-second* control to desired setting to defibrillate patient. If you want more than 200 watt-seconds, then hold in the *400 watt-seconds* button until *Watt-Sec. Meter* above reaches the desired setting.

f. Depress *buttons* on *both* paddles to fire the defibrillator.

g. Depress *Recharge* button for repeat charging and fire when needle indicator on meter reaches desired watt-seconds.

h. Turn *main power* switch *OFF* when done and return LIFEPAK/33 to *Charge Pak* and plug into power source.

i. Continuous monitoring can be done by plugging in patient cable (the paddles will not monitor if the patient cable is connected).

Figure 35   91

Fig. 35.   Attending Physician Work Schedule Memo

TO: Attending Physicians

FROM: Program Director

RE: Attending Physicians' *Final* Work Schedule

Enclosed is the Attending Physicians' FINAL Work Schedule for the period of _____. As indicated by the asterisks, there have been a number of changes in the final schedule as compared to the temporary schedule. Would you please contact me if you are involved in a change and such change is not possible, and I will make the necessary corrections. If I do not hear from you, I will assume that all dates are acceptable with your schedule.

Physicians are scheduled for laboratory evaluations as well as exercise sessions. As indicated by the enclosed schedule, on those days when a laboratory evaluation is to be conducted, your services will be needed at 4:00 p.m. in the Human Performance Laboratory. On those days when only an exercise session is conducted, your services will be needed at approximately 4:55 p.m. in the exercise area. If conflicts arise concerning your attendance for either a laboratory evaluation and/or exercise session as scheduled, please contact me at your earliest convenience so I may help make arrangements for your replacement.

Thank you for your time and consideration concerning the Cardiac Rehabilitation Program.

Fig. 36. Attending Physician Work Schedule

Date	Attending Physician	Lab Eval.	Exercise Session	Time	Place
Nov.					
2nd, Fri.	Physician No. 1		X	4:45 p.m.	Exercise Area
5th, Mon.	Physician No. 2	X	X	4:00 p.m.	Hum. Per. Lab
7th, Wed.	Physician No. 3	X	X	4:00 p.m.	Hum. Per. Lab
9th, Fri.	Physician No. 4		X	4:45 p.m.	Exercise Area
12th, Mon.	Physician No. 5	X	X	4:00 p.m.	Hum. Per. Lab
14th, Wed.	Physician No. 6		X	4:45 p.m.	Exercise Area
16th, Fri.	Physician No. 7	X	X	4:00 p.m.	Hum. Per. Lab
19th, Mon.	Physician No. 8	X	X	4:00 p.m.	Hum. Per. Lab
21st, Wed.	Physician No. 9		X	4:45 p.m.	Exercise Area
23rd, Fri.	Physician No. 10		X	4:45 p.m.	Exercise Area
26th, Mon.	Physician No. 11	X	X	4:00 p.m.	Hum. Per. Lab
28th, Wed.	Physician No. 12	X	X	4:00 p.m.	Hum. Per. Lab
30th, Fri.	Physician No. 13		X	4:45 p.m.	Exercise Area
Dec.					
3rd, Mon.	Physician No. 14	X	X	4:00 p.m.	Hum. Per. Lab
5th, Wed.	Physician No. 15	X	X	4:00 p.m.	Hum. Per. Lab
7th, Fri.	Physician No. 16	X	X	4:00 p.m.	Hum. Per. Lab
10th, Mon.	Physician No. 17		X	4:45 p.m.	Exercise Area
12th, Wed.	Physician No. 18		X	4:45 p.m.	Exercise Area
14th, Fri.	Physician No. 19		X	4:45 p.m.	Exercise Area
17th, Mon.	Physician No. 20	X	X	4:00 p.m.	Hum. Per. Lab
19th, Wed.	Physician No. 21	X	X	4:00 p.m.	Hum. Per. Lab
21st, Fri.	Physician No. 22		X	4:45 p.m.	Exercise Area

(Etc.)

Figure 37   93

Fig. 37.   Volunteer Manual

Welcome to the Cardiac Rehabilitation Program. As a volunteer, we hope that you will find the time you spend in our program rewarding, challenging and educational. It would be difficult for this program to exist without the help and dedication of volunteers. The time and effort put forth in this program is greatly appreciated, not only by the staff of the Cardiac Rehabilitation Program, but also by the participants of the program. Your greatest reward will be the personal satisfaction you receive from giving yourself and your time to someone else.

We thank you for your help. We appreciate the personal warmth and friendliness that only you as a volunteer can bring to our participants.

GENERAL INFORMATION FOR VOLUNTEERS

DRESS

1. Men—physical education shorts and t-shirts or Cardiac Rehabilitation outfits.
2. Women—physical education shorts and tops or Cardiac Rehabilitation outfits.
3. Swimming pool—conservative outfits; no tight fitting or two-piece outfits permitted. (Women who do not have a one-piece suit should wear a shirt over their suits.)
4. Cardiac Rehabilitation outfits can be purchased. For further information, contact the Program Assistants or Graduate Assistants in the program.

TIME

Report to Program Assistant at designated times as specified in the job description.

CARDIOPULMONARY RESUSCITATION (CPR)

You will be given specific responsibilities for cardiopulmonary resuscitation. Make sure you understand your responsibility. If you do not, please ask the Program Assistant in charge of the track or pool. Each month you will be required to attend a CPR education session. You will be informed of the topic and the date of the sessions by a Program Assistant.

THE EXERCISE PRESCRIPTION

Each patient is given an exercise prescription based on the results of a graded exercise test (treadmill test). The exercise prescription will be in terms of heart rate for ten seconds. Therefore, you will often notice our patients taking their heart rates. These heart rates should be taken immediately after exercise (running or calisthenics). You should know what your patient's exercise prescription is and make sure that the patient stops when he has reached his prescribed heart rate. (One beat over exercise prescription occasionally is all right.)

HEART RATE

Learn to take your pulse count accurately for ten seconds, always starting the count from zero.

The wrist (radial) pulse is the preferred site: other sites are the neck (carotid) or elbow (brachial) arteries.

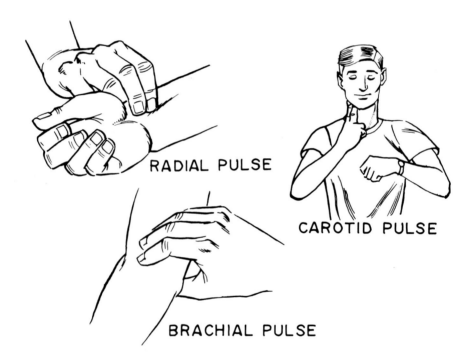

RADIAL PULSE

CAROTID PULSE

BRACHIAL PULSE

INSERVICE EDUCATION

On a rotational basis, the following inservice education programs are held for volunteers. Volunteers are required to attend these inservice programs.

1. Introduction to program (overview). Basic CPR procedures.
2. Laboratory evaluations.
3. Exercise Prescription. Review of CPR.
4. Swimming and track programs. Review of CPR.

Figure 37   95

SIGN IN PROCEDURES

All volunteers are required to sign in and include their check-in and check-out times. At the end of each month, a list will be available for volunteers which includes the sum total of hours put in by the individual volunteer.

WHAT WE EXPECT OF VOLUNTEERS, or
TEN COMMANDMENTS FOR VOLUNTEERS

VOLUNTEERS MUST BE

1. VERSED in their assignments. They must know how to perform their duties well and whom to ask for help. This requires thorough training and experience. That is why we like volunteers to work at least three (3) times a week, every week (excluding vacations).
2. OBSERVANT of little things. They must realize that it is the little "extras" that make a task a pleasure and the service appreciated.
3. LIBERAL with their neighborliness. Volunteers bring a touch of friendliness into our program—an atmosphere of "we want to" instead of "we must." However, volunteers must not select "pet" patients and ignore others. Nor can they get involved in a patient's personal and special affairs. Certainly a volunteer should avoid formality, but we believe it advisable to call patients by their surnames, "(Mr., Mrs., Ms.) _____."
4. UNDERSTANDING of patients. They must remember at all times that they are dealing with cardiac patients. Volunteers must keep themselves interested in patients, but not get themselves personally involved. If the patient insists on talking about his troubles and problems, remain interested by listening without agreeing.
5. NEAT in appearance. Good grooming for a volunteer worker includes a neat and clean gym outfit. It is preferable that you wear the designated gym outfit.
6. TACTFUL in manner. Someone has suggested that a volunteer should approach a patient as one would call on a new neighbor. The patient is the host and the volunteer the guest.
7. ETHICAL in dealings. Volunteers learn many things about patients—their families, their ailments, their treatment. This information is to be regarded as confidential. Like the tools in your kitchen, use it when needed, but return it to its "storage place" when finished.
8. EFFICIENT while serving. Volunteers must be faithful and regular in reporting for duty. When unable to come, they should notify their supervisor in time so that substitutes can be procured. While on the job, volunteers are always on the lookout for ways of serving. "Going the second mile" is characteristic of good voluntary effort.

9. REFRESHING in their contacts. One of the great assets of a volunteer is that he or she is "unofficial" in the eyes of the patient. The volunteer is a "friend" rather than a "firm." They can and should talk about things other than the patient's condition. They are a diversion from the job of getting well. The volunteer's attitude and approach can do much to create this atmosphere.

10. SOUND in mind and body. Volunteers are physically able to do the swimming, walking and running that goes with many assignments. When they have colds, they avoid contact with the patients.

DO'S, DON'TS AND NEVER NEVER'S

DO'S

1. Always sign in and out of the program.
2. Regard confidence as sacred.
3. Be friendly without being personal.
4. Be mature in your actions; act like an adult, not a teen-ager.
5. Follow instructions meticulously.

DON'TS

1. Discuss one patient with another.
2. Discuss staff members with a patient.
3. Discuss a doctor or nurse with a patient.
4. Accept personal gifts if you can avoid doing so.

NEVER NEVER'S

1. Discuss or repeat anything you have heard or observed, whether it be medical or otherwise. It is someone else's personal business.
2. Get emotionally involved.
3. Promise something you cannot fulfill.
4. Interfere with the work of professional people.
5. Smoke, chew gum or eat while on duty.

VOLUNTEER JOB DESCRIPTIONS

As a volunteer, you will be asked to work either in the swimming pool or on the track. In either situation, specific job descriptions have been made to aid volunteers in understanding their job responsibilities. The job descriptions are designated as follows:

I. Swimming pool.

A. Sheet recorders.
B. Swimming pool equipment assistants.

Figure 37   97

C. Swimming pool walkers.
D. Swimming teaching assistants.
E. Swimming assistants.

II. Track.

A. Sheet recorders.
B. Track equipment assistants.
C. Track running assistants.

I. SWIMMING POOL

A. Swimming Pool Sheet Recorders
1. Dress in locker room and report to swimming pool by 4:50 p.m.
2. Report to Exercise Leader with clipboard and sheets.
   a. Each patient has one sheet.
   b. Sheets include patient's name and exercise heart rate.
   c. The exercise heart rate is the maximal number of times the heart should beat (pulse) for ten seconds for each patient.
   d. During the exercise session patients will call out their name and heart rates for ten seconds with the number of widths they have done.
      Example: Mr. Jones will swim two widths and have a heart rate of 17. You will record 17-2 in the indicated columns.
3. You will be assigned a number of clients and will record their pulse rates on the sheets throughout the exercise session.
4. If a patient's pulse is equal to or exceeds his prescribed heart rate, you should report this to the Exercise Leader.
5. At the end of the exercise session each patient will record five consecutive heart rates. If the rates are equal to or exceed the maximum heart rate, ask the patient to stay and inform the Exercise Leader.
6. If a patient fails to record a heart rate, remind him of his failure.
7. Always refer to the patient as Mr., Mrs., Miss, or Ms.

B. Swimming Pool Equipment Assistants
1. Change in locker room and report to pool at 4:55 p.m.
2. Place mats on edge of pool. Keep mats two to three feet apart.
3. After warm-up exercises on deck have been completed, roll up mats and stand them against the wall.
4. Place marker buoys across pool.
5. Be sure that six or seven life belts are on the pool deck near the shallow end.
6. Check with pool supervisor for further duties.

C. Swimming Pool Walkers

1. Change in locker room and report to the pool by 4:55 p.m.
2. When warm-up exercises begin, stand behind patients and follow warm-up exercises. Assist any patient who is performing the exercises incorrectly.
3. When patients enter pool for further warm-up exercises, follow and again do all exercises and help those who need assistance.
4. Before walking begins, pool supervisor will assign you to a patient.
5. Go to the person and introduce yourself. Stay with that patient until all the exercises have been completed and assist if needed during the one-minute float.
6. *Remember:*
   a. A person who is walking is a new patient and should be encouraged to walk easy.
   b. We want the participants to exercise gradually, so that the next day they will not feel as if they have done anything.
   c. Patients generally walk for the first two weeks of the program.
   d. Walking is a method of easing them into the program.
   e. Each patient has an exercise heart rate. He should exercise at or below that rate. The heart rate is the number of heart beats for ten seconds.
   f. In the first week, walk two widths with the patient and then have him take his pulse rate.
   g. This can be taken below the jaw in the side of the neck or on the wrist. If you cannot take a pulse, see the pool supervisor to get proper instructions.
   h. If patients are exercising at or below their prescription rates, then during the second week they may walk four or six widths before taking their heart rates.
   i. Walking should be a heel-to-toe process.
   j. If a patient's heart rate goes above his prescribed rate, tell him to take it easy and rest a while. If the heart rate doesn't go down, inform the pool supervisor.
7. Keep patients walking in a circle. If patients seem to be bumping into each other, consult the pool supervisor.
8. Try to converse with your client—show an interest in him. This is a new experience for him and you have a great deal of influence at this stage.
9. When beginning with the patient, ask him how he feels. Ask whether he is unusually tired or has unusual pain or feelings. Consult the pool supervisor if you have any doubt, no matter how small, about the patient's condition.
10. When walking continually, find out how your client feels. Ask

Figure 37   99

whether he has any pain, numbness, soreness, or unusual feeling. Consult pool supervisor if there are problems.

11. When the patient's exercise heart rate is above his prescribed level, have the patient stop until the rate returns to normal.
12. Every few minutes, take the patient's pulse to make sure that he is reporting the correct rate.

D. Swimming Teaching Assistants
  1. Dress in locker room and report to swimming pool by 4:50 p.m.
  2. Preferably, swimming teaching assistants have attained the status of WSI (Water Safety Instructor, American Red Cross), with the ability to instruct elementary backstroke with correct whipkick.
  3. Know clients well enough to determine whether they have any previous fear of the water or knowledge of swimming.
  4. *Safety factors to be considered and stressed are:*
      a. Does patient have a safety belt on?
      b. Before pushing off from the side, watch out for people already swimming.
      c. Swim ahead of the patient so that you can get into a cross-chest carry position in the event of instability or trouble. Also, placing a hand under the patient's upper back permits guidance and promotes confidence.
      d. Avoid a head-wall collision by notifying patient before he reaches the wall.
      e. Be alert for head-head collisions.
      f. Know the patient's maximal prescribed heart rate, and notify the pool supervisor if any unusual symptoms should occur. You should have all pertinent information on the patient's performance during the walking phase of the pool program.
  5. *Aids to teaching*
      a. Have the patient get his feet wet first, so that getting the entire body wet is not so great a shock.
      b. Tell the patient to breathe normally always—he should never hold his breath. The elementary backstroke lends itself to easy breathing. (Theoretically, breath-holding initiates an increase in blood pressure.)
      c. Don't let the whole pool know what you're doing; give the patient constructive criticism about his swimming.
      d. Always try to encourage.
      e. Don't be afraid to request assistance in teaching a difficult person.
  6. Objectives in teaching the elementary backstroke
      a. To teach the patient a stroke that will allow him to swim without holding his breath.

b. To improve arm and leg coordination.

c. To teach the proper mechanics of swimming on one's back.

7. General information on the elementary backstroke

   a. Body position

     (1) The body is in a supine horizontal position.

     (2) The body is practically submerged except for the head. (Face is completely out of the water and there should be no interference with normal breathing.)

     (3) The back should be almost flat with the hips slanted down, slightly lower than the head and shoulders.

   b. Arm action

     (1) Beginning from the glide position, the hands are drawn slowly along the sides by flexing the elbows.

     (2) The hands and elbows remain close to the body throughout this movement.

     (3) At this extended position, the fingers are pointed outward, palms facing backward.

     (5) To start the propulsive phase of the elementary back stroke, the palms and inside of the arms then press simultaneously back toward the feet in a wide sweeping movement until the hands return back to the extended position.

     (6) The arm action is performed beneath the surface of the water.

   c. Leg action

     (1) In the gliding position, the legs are straight, fully extended, and together.

     (2) Start by flexing the knees and ankles so that the heels drop down and move back toward the hips. Thighs should be in line with the body and kept fairly straight.

     (3) When the heels have dropped directly below the knees, the feet are rotated so that the toes are pointed to the side. The knees are spread slightly and the feet are rotated to a position outside the knees.

     (4) Recovery is done slowly and easily to lessen resistance.

     (5) The legs are then in a position for the positive action.

     (6) Without pausing, the thrust is made by pressing backward and upward as the inside of the lower left leg and foot is pressing back against the water.

     (7) The legs finish the full extension until the feet are back into the glide position with toes pointed.

     (8) The entire movement is performed in one continuous and flowing movement that ends with the legs coming together in the extended position and the toes pointed.

   d. Breathing

     (1) The face should be out of the water at all times.

Figure 37   101

(2) Suggest that the participant breathe as normally and rhythmically as possible.

(3) Often, inhalation occurs during the recovery and exhalation during the positive action of the arm and legs.

8. Suggestions in teaching the elementary backstroke
   a. Develop within the participant a readiness for learning.
   b. Work on a ratio of one instructor to one patient. If at all possible, the instructor should remain the same throughout the learning process.
   c. Use tact and patience in teaching individuals who are unaccustomed to swimming or who have an unusual fear of the water.
   d. Use a calm, well-controlled voice, rather than an excitable one, when speaking to the patient.
   e. It is critically important to teach the patient to feel secure in the water before making any serious attempt to teach the elementary backstroke.
   f. Keep the fun in fundamentals.
   g. A demonstration is more effective than a verbal explanation.
   h. Encouragement goes a long way with patients.

E. **Swimming Assistants**
   1. Dress in locker room and report to swimming pool at 4:45 p.m.
   2. Assist in setting up equipment and warm-up exercises.
   3. You should be a strong swimmer capable of rescuing a large man if you intend to swim with the patients in the deep end.
   4. Make sure that people are swimming in a circle or an organized fashion. You may correct them.
   5. Be sure to speak to each person in your area every session. Find out how each is feeling, and just generally do some talking.
   6. Know the exercise heart rate of each person in your area, and be sure that your participant does not exceed it.
   7. Realize that these participants are more advanced—that they have been exercising longer than the walkers. Generally, they still need encouragement and advice.
   8. Be sure each participant is taking his pulse regularly. Do not let participant swim more than eight continual lengths, unless otherwise instructed.
   9. At intervals, take the pulse of anyone who continually reports an exercise heart rate that equals or exceeds his prescribed rate.

II. TRACK
   A. **Track Sheet Recorders**
      1. Dress in locker room and report to track by 4:45 p.m.
      2. Report to Exercise Leader with clipboard and sheets.
         a. Each patient has one sheet.
         b. Sheets include the patient's name and exercise heart rate.

c. The exercise heart rate is the maximal number of times the heart should beat (pulse) for ten seconds for each patient.

d. During the exercise session, patients will call out their names and heart rates for ten seconds with the number of laps they have run.

Example: Mr. Jones will run two laps and have a heart rate of 17. You will record 17-2 in the indicated columns.

3. You will be assigned a number of patients and will record their pulse rates on the sheets throughout the exercise session.

4. At the end of the exercise session, each patient will record five consecutive pulse rates. If the rates are equal to or exceed the maximal heart rate, ask the patient to stay and inform the Exercise Leader.

5. If a patient fails to record a heart rate, remind him of his failure.

6. Always refer to the patient as Mr., Mrs., Miss, or Ms.

B. Track Equipment Assistants

1. Change and report to the track at 4:55 p.m. Report to the Program Assistant.

2. Help to set up:
   a. Volleyball courts.
   b. Badminton courts.
   c. Golf driving range.
   d. Tennis courts.
   e. Stereo equipment.
   f. Blood pressure screening area.
   g. Information booth.

3. After warm-up exercises, run and walk with patients.

4. At 5:55 p.m., during final cool-down exercises, put away all of the equipment that has been set up. Have tennis nets set up on each court by 6:00.

5. Help Program Assistant whenever help is required.

C. Track Running Assistants

1. Dress in locker room and report to track at 4:45 p.m.

2. Go to assigned patient and introduce yourself.

3. When warm-up exercising begins, stand behind the patient and follow the warm-up exercises. Assist any patient who is performing the exercise incorrectly.

4. When patients start running, follow your client on the outside and slightly behind. Have patient set the pace.

5. Make sure you know the patient's exercise prescription. If the patient goes over, tell him to slow down. If he continues to disobey, report patient to Program Assistant.

6. While running, talk to the patient. Make running enjoyable, but don't forget to keep count of the laps.

Figure 37   103

7. Become familiar with the running and walking limitations for new patients and the progression each patient should be following.
8. Make sure patients are taking pulse rates immediately after exercise.
9. After 5:35, encourage participation in a lifetime activity (golf, badminton, tennis or volleyball). Some patients will prefer to run the entire hour; please respect these individual requests.
10. Participate in cool-down exercises with patients at end of exercise session.

Fig. 38. Phase I, Coronary Care Unit Protocol

1. Admit to CCU. Specify: Myocardial infarction
   - a.   Anterior wall ____
   - b.   Posterior wall ____
   - c.   Possible infarct ____
2. Record vital signs: Blood pressure, pulse, respiration q 15 min. until stable; then q 1 hour. May decrease to q 2 hours after 12 hours.
3. Administer O_2 per nasal prongs at 2 liters/min.; otherwise, ____ liters/min.
4. Administer D_5W IV at 40 ml./hour; otherwise, ____ ml./hour. Start with intravenous catheter or Teflon sheath needle if possible.
5. Attach cardiac monitor.
6. Administer lidocaine:
   - a. 50 mg. bolus stat for numerous PVCs:
     - (1) 1 PVC/8 sec. ECG sweep for three to four sweeps.
     - (2) multiple PVCs on any sweep.
     - (3) multifocal PVCs.
     - Repeat q 5 min. until controlled. If repeated doses of lidocaine are required over 30 min., start 2000 mg. of lidocaine with 500 ml. D_5W at 30 ml./hour (or 2 mg./min.). *Notify physician.*
   - b. 100 mg. bolus for ventricular tachycardia: Defibrillate electrically and give 100 mg. lidocaine for ventricular fibrillation.
7. *Notify physician stat* in case of second or third degree heart block or sinus bradycardia with rate below 45. If unable to reach physician, notify cardiologist on call or house staff member on Cardiology Service.
   - a. Titrate isoproterenol (Isuprel) 0.2 mg. in 500 ml. D_5W for second and third degree heart block with ventricular rate below 40/min.
   - b. Maintain ventricular rate at 50 to 70/min.
8. For significant drop in blood pressure:
   - a. Raise legs.
   - b. If no result, titrate phenylephrine (Neo-Synephrine) 50 mg. in 500 ml. D_5W to maintain blood pressure above 80 mm. Hg systolic.
   - c. *Notify physician stat.*
9. Record intake and output. *Notify physician if urine output is below 250 ml. in 8 hours.*
10. Diet: 1200 calories, 1 gm. sodium diet, low cholesterol.
11. Administer meperidine (Demerol), 25 mg. IV q 10 min. ×3, then q 3 hours prn.
12. Give milk of magnesia 1 oz. qd if no bowel movement.
13. Initiate in-hospital cardiac rehabilitation program at level ____.
14. Laboratory studies (cross out any not wanted):
    Day 1: SGOT, LDH, CBC, CPK, sed rate, BUN, SMA-12, urinalysis, portable chest roentgenogram, and ECG if not done previously.
    Day 2: SGOT, LDH, ECG, and chest film.

Figure 38   105

Day 3: SGOT, LDH, and ECG.

Any patient receiving diuretic agents will have determinations of Na and K every other day.

Discharge: ECG and chest film.

15. Weigh daily.
16. Volleyball for leg exercise. The ball must be placed between the patient's legs to result in tactile stimulation and prevent blood coagulation.

    (1) Primary Physician _____

    (2) House Staff Coverage _____

Fig. 39. Phase I, Ward Rehabilitation Program*

EXERCISE	WARD ACTIVITY	PATIENT EDUCATIONAL AND CRAFT ACTIVITIES
STEP 1 1. Three times daily, full passive ROM to all extremities. Each motion to be done five times. 2. Teach patient to perform active foot circles at ankles every two hours. Key Word: *myocardial infarction (M. I.)**	1. Feeding self with bed rolled up. Trunk and arms supported. 2. Partial personal care, washing face and hands (nurse should brush teeth). 3. Bedside commode.	DOCTOR'S INITIAL ____ DATE ____ 1. Initial interview and brief orientation to program.
STEP 2 1. Three times daily, assist patient in doing shoulder flexion, elbow flexion, and hip flexion and extension. Perform each motion five times. 2. Encourage foot circling. Key Word: *angina*	1. Armchair rest 20 min. two times daily, not during or immediately following meals. 2. Complete bed bath by the nurse. 3. Feeding self with bed up, trunk and arms supported. 4. Partial personal care. 5. Bedside commode.	DOCTOR'S INITIAL ____ DATE ____ 1. May read with trunk and arms supported.

Figure 39   107

STEP 3

1. Three time daily, full active ROM to all extremities while lying down. Do each motion five times.
2. Encourage foot circling.

Key Word: *atherosclerosis*

STEP 4

1. Three times daily, full active ROM to all extremities while lying down. Do each motion five times.
2. Three times daily, have patient stiffen all muscles to count of 2. Stiffen 1, 2, or 4 limbs simultaneously, depending on patient's tolerance. Count out loud. Tell patient not to hold his breath.
3. Encourage foot circling.

Key Words: *cholesterol, saturated fat, polyunsaturated fat.*

1. Feeding self in armchair with arms supported.
2. Armchair rest with meals and at bedtime, 20 min.
3. Partial personal care.
4. Complete bed bath by nurse.
5. Bathroom privileges with assistance.

1. Feeding self in armchair with arms supported.
2. Armchair rest with meals and at bedtime, 20 min.
3. Partial personal care.
4. Complete bed bath by the nurse.
5. Bathroom privileges with assistance, if necessary.

DOCTOR'S INITIAL _____ DATE _____

1. May read with trunk and arms supported.

DOCTOR'S INITIAL _____ DATE _____

1. May read with trunk and arms supported.
2. Light handcraft.

*Key words are to be utilized as discussion points with patients while they are involved in Phase I of Cardiac Rehabilitation.

EXERCISE

STEP 5

1. Three times daily, full ROM in bed at 45° with moderate resistance. Do each motion five times.
2. Introduce proper breathing techniques for exercising.
3. Encourage foot circling.

Key Word: *plaque(s)*

STEP 6

1. Three times daily, while sitting on side of bed:
   a. Full ROM of arms against resistance. Do each motion five times.
   b. Resistance to knee flexion and extension, five times.

Key Word: *coronary artery*

WARD ACTIVITY

1. Sitting ad lib.
2. Dressing, shaving, combing hair (sitting down).
3. Walking in room two times daily with assistance.
4. Bathroom privileges with assistance, if necessary.
5. Complete bed bath with minimal assistance.

1. Walk to bathroom ad lib.
2. With supervision, wash by sink sitting down.
3. Siting ad lib.
4. Dressing, shaving, combing hair (sitting down).
5. Walking in room two times daily with assistance.

PATIENT EDUCATIONAL AND CRAFT ACTIVITIES

DOCTOR'S INITIAL _____ DATE _____

1. Same as foregoing.

DOCTOR'S INITIAL _____ DATE _____

1. Introduction to home rehabilitation program:
   a. Walking
   b. Cycling

Doctor's Intitial _____

Figure 39   109

STEP 7
1. Same as foregoing.
2. Walk 50 ft. (¼ length of hall and back) at average pace.

1. Bathe in tub (must have assistance getting in and out of tub). If tub is out of room, have patient ride in wheelchair.
2. Sitting ad lib.
3. Walk to bathroom ad lib.
4. Dressing, shaving, combing hair while sitting down.

DOCTOR'S INITIAL ＿＿ DATE ＿＿
1. Instruction in early warning symptoms of a heart attack.

Key Word: *coronary thrombosis*

STEP 8
1. Three times daily, standing warm-up exercises:
   a. Arms straight out from the shoulders. Simultaneously rotate arms in big circles, five times each direction.
   b. Stand on toes ten times or abduct each leg five times.
2. May walk ½ length of hall and back two times daily with assistance, if necessary (100 ft.).

1. Same as foregoing.

DOCTOR'S INITIAL ＿＿ DATE ＿＿
1. Heart Attack: Recovery and Rehabilitation.

Key Word: *right ventricle*

EXERCISE	WARD ACTIVITY	PATIENT EDUCATIONAL AND CRAFT ACTIVITIES
		DOCTOR'S INITIAL ____ DATE ____
STEP 9	1. Walk to waiting room three times daily. May stay for 5 or 10 minutes if tolerated.	1. Living with Angina Pectoris or Living with Heart Failure.
1. Warm-up exercises three times daily:		
a. Lateral side bending, five times each side.		
b. Trunk twisting (right hand to left knee and left hand to right knee), five times each side.		
2. May walk one length of hall and back two times daily, with assistance if necessary (200 ft.).		
Key Word: *left ventricle*		
		DOCTOR'S INITIAL ____ DATE ____
STEP 10	1. Walk to waiting room two times daily—may stay 10 to 20 minutes if tolerated.	1. Relaxation Skills
1. Warm-up exercises three times daily:		
a. Lateral side-bending, ten times each side.		
b. Slight knee bends with hands on hip, ten times. Keep heels on floor.		
2. Increase walking distance; walk down one flight of stairs and take elevator up.		
Key Word: *risk factors*		

Figure 39   111

STEP 11

1. Warm-up exercises three times daily:
   a. Lateral side bending with 1-lb. weight, ten times.
   b. Standing—leg raising while leaning against wall, five times each leg.
2. Walk down one flight of stairs and take elevator up.

Key Word: *high blood pressure (hypertension)*

1. Same as foregoing.

DOCTOR'S INITIAL ____ DATE ____
1. Smoking: What Your Doctor Wants You to Know.

STEP 12

1. Warm-up exercises three times daily:
   a. Lateral side-bending with 1-lb. weight while leaning against wall, ten times each side.
   b. Leg raising, five times each leg.
   c. Trunk twisting with 1-lb. weight, five times each side.
2. Walk down one flight of stairs and take elevator up.

Key Word: *congestive heart failure*

1. Walk to waiting room ad lib.

DOCTOR'S INITIAL ____ DATE ____
1. Sex and the Heart Patient.

EXERCISE	WARD ACTIVITY	PATIENT EDUCATIONAL AND CRAFT ACTIVITIES
		DOCTOR'S INITIAL ___ DATE ___
STEP 13	1. Self-dressing in street clothes for ½ day.	1. Medications: General instructions
1. Warm-up exercises three times daily:		
a. Lateral side-bending with 2-lb. weight, ten times.		
b. Leg raising leaning against wall, ten times each.		
c. Trunk twisting with 2-lb. weight, ten times.		
Key Word: *nitroglycerin (NTG)*		
		DOCTOR'S INITIAL ___ DATE ___
STEP 14	1. Dressing in street clothes as tolerated.	1. Discharge briefing.
1. Warm-up exercises three times daily:		
a. Lateral side-bending with 2-lb. weight, ten times each side.		
b. Trunk-twisting with 2-lb. weight, ten times each side.		
c. Sit in chair, bend and touch toes ten times.		
2. Walk up one flight of stairs and then down.		
Key Word: *propranolol (Inderal)*		

Adapted from Wenger, N.K.: *Coronary Care—Rehabilitation after Myocardial Infarction.* New York, American Heart Association, 1973.

Figure 40   113

Fig. 40.   Cardiac Rehabilitation Home Program (Phase II) Manuals

I. INTRODUCTION

GROUP A. MYOCARDIAL INFARCTION (HEART ATTACK)

Heart attack is one of the most common important illnesses that beset men and women of your age and even younger. Although every case is individual, there is a fairly standard procedure for getting people in your condition back on their feet. The following paragraphs explain how this can best be done.

First, we tell you what has happened—what has been going on inside you. Then it will be easier for you to understand our plans for your recovery, and easier for you to help us carry them out.

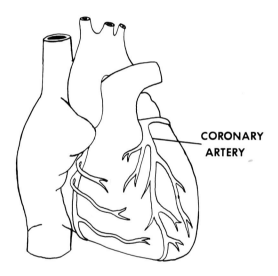

CORONARY
ARTERY

The Coronary Arteries. Actually, the heart attack that you had is not primarily a disease of the heart muscle. It is really the result of a condition in the arteries—the coronary arteries—which supply the heart muscle with blood.

The heart muscle, or myocardium as it is called, is so thick and strong and constantly active day and night that it needs its own rich blood supply. The blood that simply flows through the chambers of the heart does not supply blood to the heart muscle itself.

Therefore in the development of the human heart, an extensive network of arteries has grown out from two main trunks, the right and the left coronary arteries. These main coronary arteries branch in somewhat the same manner as a tree. Every branch is smaller than the main trunk, and each one soon subdivides into smaller branches. These in turn divide into still smaller ones which are like very tiny twigs. Every portion of the heart, no matter how small, is supplied with blood and oxygen through this system of coronary arteries.

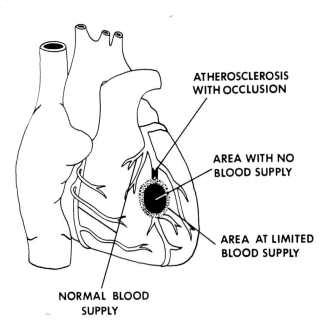

ATHEROSCLEROSIS WITH OCCLUSION

AREA WITH NO BLOOD SUPPLY

AREA AT LIMITED BLOOD SUPPLY

NORMAL BLOOD SUPPLY

Atherosclerosis. Over a period of years these coronary arteries were setting the stage for your heart attack through the gradual development of atherosclerosis. This is a form of arteriosclerosis, which is usually known to laymen as hardening of the arteries. Atherosclerosis leads to a thickening as well as a hardening of the walls of arteries. The process usually begins with the deposit of fatty material on the inner lining of the arterial wall; each individual deposit is known as an atheroma.

As more and more of these deposits are formed and increase in size, they gradually narrow the channel through which the blood flows. This happens in much the same way as deposits of rust clog a water pipe. This process leads to roughening of the lining of the artery, which is normally smooth and glistening. Some sections of the arteries may remain largely unaffected, while other sections nearby may be altered greatly.

Many people with advanced and widespread changes in their coronary arteries give no evidence of artery disease throughout a long and active life. Many such people die at 75 or 80 years of age from some condition not related to the heart: malignant tumors, infections, accidents. The reason

Figure 40   115

why these people continue living without symptoms of heart disease is that enough blood still flows through the coronary arteries to provide nourishment and energy for the heart muscle.

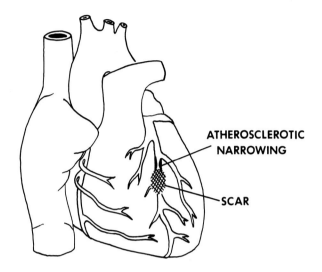

Myocardial Infarction. In your case, the atherosclerotic process has critically narrowed a branch of a coronary artery. This narrowing prevented an adequate flow of blood to part of your heart muscle, a section perhaps the size of an almond. This part of the muscle began to ache; that was the pain you felt. You had just had a heart attack (myocardial infarction).

Gradually, the fibers of this small portion of muscle stopped contracting. They became swollen and died, and the pain slowly went away. This portion of heart muscle actually suffered an acute injury. Like acute injuries in other tissues of the body, it requires time for its healing.

The Healing Process. Your body began the healing process by sending "wrecking cells" (leukocytes) to clear away the muscle fibers that were no longer able to contract. This has to be done before the tissue can heal and form a strong scar. The clearing-away process takes about a week or a little longer. During this time you may have a slight fever.

At the end of the first week you may feel perfectly well; but actually that injured portion of your heart forms a weak area in the muscle wall. Until a scar forms and toughens, you must limit your activity.

Meanwhile other repair work goes on. Other arterial branches enlarged and new branches began to form to bring a supply of blood to the area around the injury. These new branches are known as the "collateral circulation;" they often play an important part in the healing process.

We watched the mending process by making certain blood tests, by examining your electrocardiograms and chest x-ray pictures, by taking your pulse and blood pressure frequently, and by noting any symptoms that you reported to us.

As the process of healing progressed you were started through a program of mild, but gradually progressive exercises. This was designed to prevent the process of deconditioning associated with your lack of physical activity but mild enough not to cause further muscle damage.

You might want to think of your injury as similar in some respects to a bone fracture in your leg. Even if a large bone were fractured, you would be comfortable within several days, but the bone could not support your weight until the injury had healed solidly.

The injury to your heart is going to leave a small scar; this will probably be formed within the first two or three weeks. During the second month, the scar should become firm and healing would be completed.

Both bone fractures and injuries to the heart vary in their severity and in the length of time required for healing, and, as with any kind of healing process, some people mend faster than others. That is why doctors would rather not estimate in advance exactly when you will leave the hospital and exactly when you will be at work again. But just as a bone fracture heals with care and time, so, if all goes well, several weeks should be enough to get you fully back into normal activity again—and that means back to your job.

We have every reason to believe that you will resume your regular life, although we *may* have to ask that you reduce some of your more strenuous physical activities.

It is current opinion that a perfectly firm, well-healed scar may cause no trouble for the remainder of a long life. But that optimism can be overdone and lead to overconfidence and carelessness. In a few cases, complications may delay the healing process.

Remember that heart attacks vary greatly in severity, and the treatment also may vary. Some patients may have considerable discomfort for a number of days, while others may have none after the first day. Some may be given oxygen for five or six days or even longer, and some may not require oxygen at all. Some receive drugs known as anticoagulants, but doctors do not necessarily prescribe these for all patients.

Watching for Symptoms. You and your family should be aware of possible future symptoms, both important and trivial.

Doctors realize that sensitive people may become heart-conscious after recovering from a heart attack, and may be unnecessarily worried by symptoms of little or no importance, such as fatigue, palpitation, or heartburn. On the other hand, symptoms such as unusual shortness of breath or discomfort behind the breastbone might indicate additional problems and should be reported to your doctor.

Figure 40   117

No matter how slight your symptoms are, you are encouraged to report to your doctor any discomfort and all symptoms that are causing anxiety. During normal office hours call your physician directly. On weekends, holidays or evenings, call the emergency department of the hospital.

The majority of persons who recover from a heart attack are able to walk, play golf, fish, and engage in similar activities without trouble. Many doctors believe that such exercises in moderation are beneficial rather than harmful, provided they do not cause symptoms.

What Caused Your Heart Attack? Doctors do not yet know exactly what causes those changes in arteries known as atherosclerosis. There is fairly general agreement that probably many different factors are responsible, such as heredity, obesity, high blood pressure, smoking, diabetes, and others that are related in some way to atherosclerosis. Although the evidence is incomplete, diet in general and fats in particular cannot be ruled out of the heart disease picture. Some authorities believe that the kind and amount of fat in the diet may be related in some way to the development of atherosclerosis in the coronary arteries.

Once a coronary artery has become narrowed as a result of atherosclerosis, a clot or thrombus may form and close the artery. When this happens, it is not known why the thrombus forms just at the time it did.

Although the term "coronary thrombosis" is often used interchangeably with the term heart attack, it should be emphasized that the formation of a thrombus is not the only way in which an artery may be closed. In a great many cases an artery is closed as a result of a steady increase in the size of the atheromas—the fatty deposits on the inner lining of the artery wall. In many cases the closure is thought to be brought about by small hemorrhages in the wall of the artery.

Could Your Heart Attack Have Been Prevented? In all probability, the intensive research now going on will lead us some day to a full knowledge of the fundamental cause or causes of atherosclerosis. When this knowledge is available, we may be able to modify or prevent atherosclerosis and thus reduce or abolish heart attacks. Today we are able to recognize coronary atherosclerosis when it has announced its presence by an actual heart attack, by the symptom known as angina pectoris, by changes in the electrocardiogram, or with certain blood tests. New techniques are now being explored which may make it possible to recognize coronary atherosclerosis in apparently well persons and thus permit early treatment in the hope of modifying the condition.

In the following sections a program of activity to be followed during the next eight weeks will be covered. This program is designed to gradually return you to your pre-infarction level of physical activity. In fact, if you follow this program you may find that your level of physical conditioning is better than it was before your heart attack. Strict adherence to these procedures will ensure your rapid recovery. A list of tips to save your heart work is included for your information. Also, a home dietary program is included to help you lower the saturated fats and cholesterol in your diet.

GROUP B. CORONARY BYPASS SURGERY

Congratulations on your recovery after your coronary bypass surgery. You have passed the initial and most dangerous stages of the operation, and further recovery should proceed smoothly and steadily.

Your operation is called "bypass surgery" because new blood vessels have been attached to your heart to bypass blocked areas in your coronary arteries. The doctors were able to locate the blocked areas by doing the heart catheterization study before the surgery. Hopefully the beneficial effects of the bypass grafts will be long-lasting. Studies conducted by us and others indicate that in approximately eight or nine out of ten such operations, the new blood vessels remain open and functioning after surgery. Although it is possible that the arteriosclerosis problem that caused your heart trouble could recur in other coronary arteries or even in the bypass grafts themselves, such an event is rare in our experience, especially if the patient follows advice regarding diet, exercise, medication, and smoking.

The drawing shows a heart with two bypass grafts. One is a saphenous vein graft, which has been taken from the leg; the other is an internal mammary artery graft, which is taken from under the ribs.

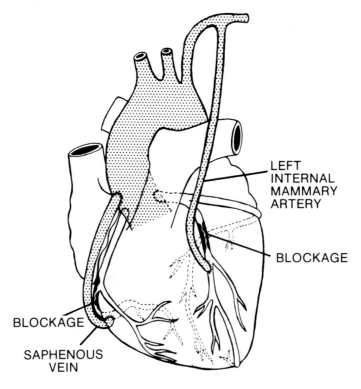

Figure 40   119

Recovery. Your operation has been a major one, about as serious as any that doctors can perform today. For this reason, recovery is slow, and you will feel tired for a period of four to six weeks, which is probably longer than you expected. Along with this you will probably feel depressed or "down." These two feelings, fatigue and depression, are almost natural occurrences following major surgery. Because of these reactions it is wise to follow an exercise program along with the other advice we outline here. The total recovery period, which extends from the time of surgery until you can return to work and thoroughly enjoy life again, usually lies somewhere between six weeks and three months.

Everyone experiences chest pain and aching in and around the incision. It usually lasts six weeks to three months, generally as long as the recovery period. The best treatment for this is time, but pain medication (Darvon or Tylenol) often provides a welcome relief. If other pains occur during your recovery that are different from your incision pain, tell your doctor.

GROUP C. HEART VALVE REPLACEMENT SURGERY

Congratulations on your recovery after your valve replacement surgery. You have passed the initial and most dangerous stages of the operation, and further recovery should proceed smoothly and steadily.

Heart valve replacement surgery began about 20 years ago. Since that time, scientists and surgeons have been improving the operation and the artificial valves themselves, so that now the entire procedure is regarded as safe and standard.

Your new valve, whether it is a "pig" valve or a mechanical type, is durable and reliable, a fact learned from hundreds of hours of testing and from an accumulation of many years of experience in patients. If your heart had suffered significant fatigue and damage before your valve surgery, there may be some lasting damage, even though the valve itself has been repaired. Often, the seriousness of the residual damage can only be revealed by gauging the extent of your recovery following surgery. During this prolonged recovery period your doctor will help all he can with medications and advice and he will be continually on the lookout for signs of improvement in your condition, just as you will.

Recovery. Your operation has been a major one, about as serious as any that doctors can perform today. For this reason the recovery is slow and you will probably continue to feel tired and "run down" for two to three months following the surgery. Along with this you will probably feel some mild or moderate depression. These two feelings, fatigue and depression, are almost natural occurrences following major surgery, particularly surgery on the heart. Because of these feelings you will need a program of rehabilitation. Such a program, which appears on the following pages, may become the key to your return to a normal life.

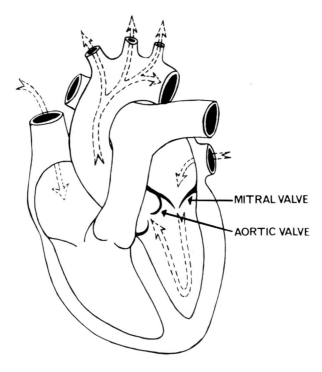

MITRAL VALVE

AORTIC VALVE

Mechanical Valve
(Björk)

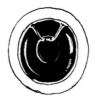

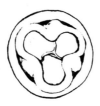

Porcine Valve
(Pig)

Figure 40 121

Everyone experiences some degree of aching pain in the incision, which usually lasts about six weeks to three months. The best treatment for this is time, but Darvon or Tylenol often provides a welcome relief. Usually, you should not take aspirin, because aspirin interferes with the drug warfarin, which is an anticoagulant medicine that most valve replacement patients require.

Patients frequently ask "when can I go back to work?" The standard answer is "about three months after the surgery." Naturally, this may be longer for some patients, less for others, depending on the severity of the underlying heart weakness and the degree of exertion required for the job.

II. SPECIAL INFORMATION AND ADVICE

A. GOING HOME

The ride home should be in a car; an ambulance is seldom necessary. Do not plan to drive yourself, and if the trip is more than an hour, plan to stop, get out of the car and walk a little so blood does not stagnate in your legs. Also, if the ride is a long one, plan to sit in the back seat with a pillow so you can lie back and rest.

B. DAILY ACTIVITIES AT HOME

Group A
1. *General Activities*
   a. *Eat three or four meals a day.* Each should contain about the same amount of food. Don't eat very large meals and eat slowly—don't rush.
   b. *Avoid tension.* Try to avoid situations, people and topics of conversation that upset you (make you tense or angry). Your heart works harder when you are angry, tense, or afraid.
   c. *Avoid being in very cold or very hot temperatures.* In the summertime, plan your outdoor activity during the cool of the day. The heat makes the heart work faster. Also, avoid chilling. If you go out on a very cold, windy day, cover your mouth and nose with a handkerchief or mask and don't take breaths of cold air.
   d. *Space your activities* to allow time for your heart to rest.
      (1) Plan your day's and week's work. Spread out harder tasks; alternate an easy task with a hard one.
      (2) If you get tired, stop and rest for 15 to 30 minutes, no matter what you are doing. Don't push yourself to clip the hedges, to mow all the grass or to watch the last 45 minutes of that T.V. show.

(3) Space your activities. Don't try to do all your chores in the morning; do some in the afternoon and some in the evening. Rest in between.

(4) Try not to hurry. Plan your day so that you can get everything done without getting tense and hurried. Don't feel you must rush to complete the job in a short time.

(5) Plan a 20- to 30-minute rest period at least twice a day, once in the morning and once in the afternoon. You don't have to go to bed—just rest.

(6) Every night, sleep the number of hours that you usually slept before your heart attack. Try to get at least six to eight hours of sleep. Do not stay up very late one night and "catch up" the next. However, if you do plan to stay up late, take a nap beforehand.

(7) Working with your arms above your shoulders is harder on your heart than working with them below shoulder level. Have someone rearrange your cabinets so that things you use often are at or below waist level. If you must have things in high cabinets, place those articles you use most often in the front. Avoid washing windows, hanging clothes on the line and reaching for things above your shoulder level.

2. *The First Two Weeks*

For the first weeks at home, continue to be as active as you were on the last day in the hospital. You can do the following things:

a. Get up and get dressed every day.

b. Walk daily. Walk as much as you were walking in the hospital. You may walk outside when the weather is nice, but walk on level ground. Follow the exercise program outlined in section four of this booklet. Plan where you will walk before you go. Avoid steps and hills—they make your heart work harder than walking on the level ground. Avoid walking against the wind because your heart works harder and beats faster then. In the winter, walk in late morning or early afternoon, during the warmest part of the day. In the summer, do your walking in the morning or evening when it is cool. Walk after a rest period or when you're not already tired from another activity. If you have chest discomfort or shortness of breath, stop and sit down on the steps or curb, take nitroglycerin if you have some, and wait until you feel OK. Tell your doctor about this pain when you see him again.

c. If your bedroom is up a flight of stairs, your doctor may suggest that you climb the stairs only once a day, and that you take only a few steps at a time and stop to rest.

d. Avoid doing anything that tenses your body, such as:

(1) straining when having a bowel movement (ask your doctor about a laxative)

Figure 40   123

(2) lifting anything heavy—children, groceries, or suitcases

(3) pushing or pulling anything heavy

(4) trying to open a stuck window or unscrew a stuck jar lid

e. Activities *you can do*:

   (1) cook one meal a day

   (2) wash dishes and clean up after another meal

   (3) tidy up the bed but not change the sheets

   (4) wash clothes—put them in the washer but have *someone else* pull them out, carry them, and hang them on the line

   (5) talk with friends as long as they don't tire you

   (6) walk on flat surfaces

   (7) shave and shower

   (8) shoot pool

   (9) throw softball (underhand)

  (10) ride in car (not driving)

  (11) go to relaxing movie or out to dinner (without cocktail)

  (12) go to grocery store with wife or husband

  (13) knit or crochet

f. Activities *you should not do:*

   (1) vacuum

   (2) sweep

   (3) heavy cleaning

   (4) drive

   (5) lift weights or do other isometrics

   (6) rake leaves, garden, pull weeds

   (7) hoe

   (8) work in attic or basement

   (9) wash car

  (10) play golf or tennis

  (11) watch excitable TV or movie

  (12) play basketball or football

  (13) ride a bike

  (14) go bowling

  (15) shovel snow or push snowblower

  (16) walk in temperatures below 20°F.

You may be able to do these things after you have been home
_____. Check with your doctor.

3. *After the First Two Weeks*

  a. You may go to church.

  b. You may go to grocery store for a few things.

  c. Ask your doctor when you may

    drive the car _____

    return to work _____

    go fishing _____

    go to the movies _____

go to a ball game _____

roll up your hair _____

   d. You may cut the lawn with a self-propelled mower or riding mower. Do this activity with care and in cool weather.

   e. When your doctor says you may go back to work, try to arrange to go back part time at first and then slowly increase your working time.

You may have other questions about your activities, diet, medications or illness. If you do, please feel free to ask us.

 4. *General Advice*

   a. If you develop pain, numbness, or shortness of breath, stop what you are doing, take your nitroglycerin if your doctor gave you some, and rest for several minutes. When the discomfort disappears, continue what you were doing but at a slower rate.

   b. Try to follow your fat-controlled diet. It is an important part of the doctor's plan for helping to reduce your blood cholesterol.

   c. Regular coffee with caffeine will increase the heart rate. One to two cups per day is all right unless your doctor states otherwise. Decaffeinated coffee (for example, Sanka) is good to use if you want to drink more than one or two cups.

   d. To protect your heart take a daily walk. A program of progressive exercise through walking is included in section four of this booklet and should be followed.

   e. Continue the physical therapy exercises started in the hospital until you return to normal activity. You should do these exercises prior to your walking program.

   f. After a meal, your heart is already working to help your body digest your food. Therefore, rest for an hour after eating before doing any heavy exercise.

   g. Stop smoking cigarettes. Smoking is bad for your lungs and your heart. Smoking cigarettes increases your chance of having another heart attack.

   h. Your doctor says you may have _____ ounces of liquor a day. Never drink enough liquor, beer, or wine to become drunk.

   i. Check with your doctor before you take a long trip. He will probably want you to wait for at least six weeks before you take a long car trip. When you go, stop every two hours and walk around—this will help prevent clots from forming in your lower legs. Be sure to check with your doctor before going to the mountains or to a place that is very hot and humid. Airplane trips are usually permitted one month after discharge.

   j. Your doctor says that you may have sexual relations _____ days after discharge. As with other activities or exercise, you should not engage in sexual activities if:

Figure 40   125

(1) you are tired (take a 30-minute nap first)

(2) you have just eaten a heavy meal

(3) you have been drinking

(4) you are angry with your mate

(5) the temperature of the room is uncomfortably warm or cool.

If you begin to have chest discomfort while having relations, STOP. The next time, try taking nitroglycerin before having relations. Remember that it is normal for your heart to beat faster and your breathing to speed up while you are having relations. Your heart beat and breathing should slow down and return to normal shortly afterward.

k. Notify your doctor immediately if you have:

(1) Heavy pressure or squeezing pain in the chest, which may spread to the shoulder, arm, neck or jaw, and is not relieved in 15 minutes by resting and/or nitroglycerin.

(2) increased shortness of breath

(3) unusual tiredness

(4) swelling of feet and ankles

(5) fainting

(6) very slow or rapid heart rate

Groups B and C

Driving

Avoid driving your car for one month after your surgery. Because of weakness, fatigue, or discomfort, your reaction time may be slow. Extended automobile trips are not advised, but if unavoidable, plan to stop the car hourly and walk around to help the circulation in your legs.

Housework

You should not plan to resume housework duties until two to three months after your surgery. However, after one month the following activities are reasonable:

Setting and clearing the table.

Assisting with meal preparation.

Dusting, light sweeping.

Activities such as raking, vacuuming, moving furniture, or lifting objects over 10 lbs. should be avoided until two months after the surgery.

Sex

Sexual activity may be resumed when you feel so inclined. Avoid over-exertion during and soon afterward.

Stairs

Climbing stairs takes more energy than walking or bicycling. You may use stairs, but go slowly at first. Stop or sit down in the middle if you become very tired, short of breath, or have pain.

Rest

Plan two 20- to 30-minute rest periods each day during the first two weeks at home. Plan eight to ten hours of sleep each night.

III. EXERCISE PROGRAM

Your recovery will be faster and better if you follow our progressive exercise program. The purpose of the program is twofold:
1. To recondition your muscles and other organs and thereby regain the tone and efficiency they had before your heart attack or surgery.
2. To help you establish an exercise habit which we hope you will continue, as we believe this can reduce your risk of recurrence of heart disease.

WALKING

It is not necessary for you to do strenuous activity or high intensity work such as jogging to accomplish our purpose. As a matter of fact, jogging in your situation could be harmful. Low intensity daily work such as walking is all that is needed for an eight-week period to significantly increase your fitness level. Because of the lower work level, the walk workout should be done *daily*. Two or three times a week at this caloric load is not frequent enough to produce positive changes.

Do not jog until this two-month phase of your conditioning program has been completed, and only then if recommended by your physician. At the completion of your rehabilitation program—eight weeks of exercise—you will be re-evaluated and given a graded exercise test prior to your returning to work and/or entering a more advanced exercise program.

To achieve maximal benefit from your beginning fitness program and to help evaluate your progress, the following is recommended:
1. *Keep a daily record.* This would involve preparing a simple chart of the date, the distance covered, the amount of time of continual walking, 10-second pulse count at the end of the walk, and any symptoms or comments you want to add. Fill this chart in every day and bring it with you on your next clinic visit.
2. *Walking should be continual and rhythmic.* Swing your arms and stride along at an even, rhythmic pace. Do not stroll along and do not stop unless necessary. Use loose-fitting clothing and comfortable shoes.
3. If your *heart rate* at the end of your walk is greater than 114 beats per minute (19 beats per 10 seconds), decrease the speed of your walk and the distance covered. Phone your physician if your heart rate after exercise is consistently over this level.
4. *Keep active during the day.* Develop better movement habits. Begin to think in terms of activity. *Sit less—move more!!!*

Figure 40   127

5. Remember that *diet control* (restricted dietary fats and proper body weight), a controlled and guided *exercise program* and *abstinence from tobacco* will significantly improve your fitness level and your entire cardiovascular system.
6. If you develop any of the following symptoms during or after your daily walk, report to your physician.
   a. Excessive fatigue
   b. Any unusual joint, muscle, or ligament problem
   c. Chest pain
   d. Pain in the teeth, jaw, arms, or ears
   e. Light-headedness or dizziness
   f. Irregularity of the pulse
   g. Nausea and/or vomiting
   h. Headache
   i. Pulse rate over 19 beats per 10 seconds at end of your exercise if decreasing speed and distance hasn't lowered your pulse rate below this level.
   j. Shortness of breath
7. Do not walk immediately after meals—wait at least ½ hour.
8. Walk on level surfaces.
9. Continue the warm-up exercises you performed on the final day of your hospitalization. Do these exercises every day, two times a day, for the duration of this eight-week exercise program. The best time is before and immediately following your walking session.
10. Don't walk outside as an exercise session when it is colder than 20°F above zero.

Warm-Up Exercises
   1. Side-Bending:
   Stand up straight with arms hanging at sides. Bend at waist, reaching down side of leg toward your knees. Repeat ten times to each side with a 2-pound weight in each hand.
   2. Knee Touches:
   Bend forward. Touch right hand to left knee. Stand up straight. Bend and touch left hand to right knee. Come up straight. Repeat this ten times with a 2-pound weight in each hand.
   3. Sitting Toe Touches:
   Sit in chair, keeping feet on floor, bend at waist and touch fingers to toes. Sit up again. Repeat ten times. *Do not use a weight with this exercise.*

Progressive Walk Schedule
   1. *First Two Weeks.*
      a. Progressively increase your walking distance on a daily basis. The first day begin with walking one block out and one block back. Progressively increase the distance by two blocks a day to a total of

five blocks out and five blocks back. You should be walking a total of ten blocks by the fifth day of the program. This walking distance should be maintained for an additional nine days.

b. Continue walking this distance for the two-week period, unless adverse symptoms develop or the pulse exceeds 114 beats per minute (19 beats per 10 seconds). If the pulse rate is below 114 beats at the end of each daily walk go on to the next level after the two weeks of exercise. If the pulse rate is 114 per minute or over, contact your primary physician.

c. There are approximately 140 yards in one block.

2. *Third and Fourth Weeks.*

   a. Measure a ¾-mile distance.
   b. Cover this distance 20 minutes out and 20 minutes back.
   c. Total distance is 1½ miles in 40 minutes.
   d. Continue walking this distance for the entire two-week period unless adverse symptoms develop or the pulse exceeds 114 beats per minute (19 beats per 10 seconds).
   e. If the pulse rate is below 114 per minute at the end of each daily walk, go on to the next level after two weeks of exercise. If the pulse rate is 114 per minute or over, contact your primary physician.
   f. There are approximately 12 blocks in a mile.

3. *Fifth and Sixth Weeks.*

   a. Measure a one-mile distance.
   b. Cover this distance 30 minutes out and 30 minutes back.
   c. Total distance is two miles in 60 minutes.
   d. Continue walking this distance for the entire two-week period, unless adverse symptoms develop or pulse exceeds 114 beats per minute (19 beats per 10 seconds).
   e. If the pulse rate is below 114 per minute at the end of each daily walk, go on to the next level after two weeks of exercise. If the pulse is 114 per minute or over, contact your primary physician.

4. *Seventh and Eighth Weeks.*

   a. Measure a 1½-mile distance.
   b. Cover this distance 36 minutes out and 36 minutes back.
   c. Total distance is three miles in 72 minutes.
   d. If the pulse is below 114 per minute at the end of each daily walk, continue at this level for a two-week period (19 beats per 10 seconds).
   e. If the pulse is 114 per minute or over, contact your primary physician.

Upon completion of this exercise program, you will be scheduled for a graded exercise test (GXT). Based on the results of this test, specific recommendations regarding your activity and work will be made.

Figure 40   129

This program is designed to return you in a stepwise fashion to full activity. If you have difficulty understanding these instructions, please feel free to contact your primary physician.

BICYCLING

Instead of a walking program, some patients prefer a bicycling program, which will accomplish the same purpose. Bicycles are available for rent or purchase from various outlets.

Do not exceed this exercise prescription until you have completed the two-month phase of your conditioning program. At the completion of this two-month period, your doctor will arrange an exercise test to determine how you should proceed with activity and exercise.

To achieve maximal benefit from your bicycling program, we recommend the following:

1. Keep a daily record. This would involve preparing a simple chart of the date, total time of continual bicycling, 10-second pulse count at rest and end of warm-up period, during exercise, and at the end of cool-down period, and any symptoms or comments you may want to add. Fill this chart in every day and bring it with you on your next visit.
2. *Bicycling should be continual and rhythmic.* Relax, use a light comfortable grip on the handle, and ride at an even, rhythmic pace at 50 pedal revolutions per minute. Do not stop unless necessary. Wear light, loose-fitting clothing and comfortable shoes.
3. *Bicycle seat adjustment.* Adjust the seat so that one leg is fully extended when the pedal is in the down position or at the bottom of a revolution.
4. If your heart rate at any time during your bicycling is greater than 114 beats per minute (19 beats per 10 seconds), decrease the resistance on your bike and maintain the pedal speed at 50 revolutions per minute. Phone your physician if your heart rate is consistently over this.
5. *Keep active during the day.* Develop better movement habits. Begin to think in terms of activity. *Sit less—move more!!!!!*
6. Remember that *diet control* (restricted dietary fats and proper body weight), a controlled and guided *exercise program*, and *abstinence from tobacco* will significantly improve your fitness level and your entire cardiovascular system.
7. If you develop any of the following symptoms during or after your daily bicycle exercise, report to your physician.
   a. Excessive fatigue.
   b. Any unusual joint, muscle, or ligament problems.
   c. Chest pain.
   d. Pain in the teeth, jaw, arms, or ears.
   e. Light-headedness or dizziness.
   f. Irregularity of the pulse.

    g. Nausea and/or vomiting.

    h. Headache.

    i. Pulse rate over 19 per 10 seconds at the end of your exercise.

    j. Shortness of breath.

8. Do not bicycle immediately after meals—wait at least ½ hour.

9. Continue the warm-up exercises you performed on the final day of your hospitalization. These exercises are to be done every day, twice a day, for the two-month period.

Warm-Up Exercises

1. Side-Bending:

Stand up straight with arms hanging at sides. Bend at waist, reaching down side of leg toward your knees. Repeat ten times to each side with a 2-pound weight in each hand.

2. Knee Touches:

Bend forward. Touch right hand to left knee. Stand up straight. Bend and touch left hand to right knee. Come up straight. Repeat this ten times with a 2-pound weight in each hand.

3. Sitting Toe Touches:

Sit in chair, keeping feet on floor, bend at waist and touch fingers to toes. Sit up again. Repeat ten times. *Do not use a weight with his exercise.*

Bicycle Exercise Description.

1. Take a resting heart rate before starting your exercises (sitting).

2. Do your warm-up exercises, including side-bending, knee touches, and sitting toe touches.

3. Do your bicycle warm-ups according to your prescription and immediately record a 10-second heart rate.

4. Readjust your resistance to your prescribed exercise program and maintain pedal speed at 50 RPM. Remember, heart rate should not exceed 114 beats per minute (19 beats per 10 seconds).

5. Continue to work at this level, recording the heart rate at prescribed times.

6. Cool down by decreasing resistance to 0. Remember to maintain pedal speed at 50 RPM.

7. Immediately following cool-down, record your heart rate.

During this exercise program, you will be scheduled for an exercise prescription check after two and four weeks. Based on the results of these checks, specific recommendations regarding your bicycle exercise program will be made. After the completion of this eight-week exercise program, you will be scheduled for a graded exercise test (GXT). At this time, specific recommendations regarding your activity and work will be made.

This program is designed to return you in a stepwise fashion to full

Figure 40   131

activity. If you have difficulty understanding these instructions, please feel free to contact your primary physician.

IV. HOME DIETARY PROGRAM

GROUPS A, B

Following a heart attack or coronary artery bypass surgery, we believe it is wise to follow a low fat, low cholesterol diet. There is no guarantee that this will prevent further fat and cholesterol deposits in your arteries, but for almost everyone it will be a help in that direction. If your doctors think you should be on a more specialized diet this will be made clear by them and the dietician before you leave the hospital.

General Advice

Every day, select foods from each of the basic food groups in lists 1 through 5 and follow the recommendations for the number and size of servings. These foods are nutritious as well as low in saturated fats and cholesterol.

List 1: Fish, Poultry, Meat, Dried Beans and Peas, Nuts, Eggs

One serving is 3 ounces cooked weight of meat (not including bone or fat) or 3 ounces of a vegetable listed here. Use two or more servings daily. Prepare by baking, broiling, roasting or stewing. Discard fat that cooks out of meat.

1. *Approved Foods:*
    a. Chicken, turkey, veal, fish
    b. Nuts, dried beans, and peas are high in vegetable protein and may be used in place of meat occasionally.
    c. Egg whites
2. *Foods with Restrictions*
    a. Lean cuts of beef, lamb, pork, rabbit.
    b. Shellfish (except shrimp), organ meats (limit either to one serving a week).
    c. Egg yolks (limit to three a week).
3. *Foods To Be Avoided:*
    a. Duck, goose
    b. Shrimp
    c. Heavily marbled and fatty meats, such as spare ribs, frankfurters, sausage, bacon or luncheon meats.

List 2: Bread and Cereals (Whole Grain, Enriched or Restored)

One serving of bread is one slice. One serving of cereal is ½ cup cooked or ¾ cup dry. Eat four or more servings daily.

1. *Approved Foods:*
    a. Breads made with a minimum of saturated fat, such as white enriched, whole wheat, English muffins, French bread, Italian bread, pumpernickel bread, oatmeal bread, and rye bread.

   b. Biscuits, muffins and griddle cakes made at home, using an allowed liquid oil as shortening.
   c. Cereals (hot and cold), rice, melba toast
   d. Pasta: macaroni, noodles (except egg noodles), spaghetti
2. *Foods To Be Avoided:*
   a. Butter rolls, commercial biscuits, muffins, donuts, sweet rolls, cakes, crackers, egg bread, cheese bread, commercial mixes containing dried eggs and whole milk.

List 3: Milk Products

One serving is 8 ounces. Adults need two or more cups of skimmed milk (fortified with vitamins A and D) per day.

1. *Approved Foods:*
   a. Fortified skimmed (nonfat) milk and fortified skimmed milk powder, 1% butterfat milk.
   b. Buttermilk made from skimmed milk.
   c. Yogurt made from skimmed milk.
   d. Canned evaporated skimmed milk.
   e. Cocoa made with skimmed or 1% butterfat milk.
   f. Cheese made from skimmed or partially skimmed milk, such as cottage cheese; farmer's, baker's, hoop cheese; mozzarella and sapsago cheeses made with partially skimmed milk, corn oil cheeses.
2. *Foods with Restrictions:*
   a. Low fat or 2% butterfat milk
   b. Low-fat yogurt
   c. Chocolate skimmed milk, ice milk
   d. Nondairy cream substitutes
3. *Foods To Be Avoided:*
   a. Canned whole milk, whole milk, chocolate milk, ice cream
   b. All creams including sour, half and half, whipped
   c. Whole milk yogurt
   d. Cheese made from cream of whole milk
   e. Butter

List 4: Fats and Oils (Polyunsaturated)

One serving is 1 teaspoon. Use 6 to 12 servings daily. Polyunsaturated fats are always of plant origin. They are thought to lower blood cholesterol. Saturated fats are *usually* of animal origin. They are thought to raise blood cholesterol.

1. *Approved Foods:*
   a. Margarines, liquid oil shortenings, salad dressings and mayonnaise containing any of these polyunsaturated vegetable oils: Corn, cottonseed, safflower, sesame seed, soybean, sunflower seed.

Figure 40   133

Margarines and other products high in polyunsaturates can usually be identified by their label, which lists a recommended *liquid* vegetable oil as the first ingredient and one or more partially hydrogenated vegetable oils as additional ingredients.

2. *Foods with Restrictions:*
   a. Peanut oil and olive oil may be used occasionally for flavor.
3. *Foods To Be Avoided:*
   a. Butter, lard, salt pork fat, meat fat
   b. Chocolate
   c. Completely hydrogenated margarines and vegetable shortenings

List 5: Vegetables and Fruits

One serving is ½ cup. Use four or more servings daily. Eat in salads, main dishes, snacks, and desserts.

1. *Approved Foods:*
   a. For Vitamin A eat carrots, broccoli, sweet potatoes, deep yellow squash, cantaloupe, peaches and apricots.
   b. For Vitamin C eat oranges, grapefruit, strawberries, melons, cabbage, potatoes, tomatoes, broccoli, brussels sprouts, cauliflower, red and green peppers.
2. *Foods with Restrictions:*
   a. If you must limit your calories to control your weight, use fresh or unsweetened frozen or canned fruit or unsweetened fruit juices.
   b. If you need to gain weight, you may want to add desserts such as flavored gelatin, skim milk pudding or angel food cake to your meals.
3. *Foods To Be Avoided:*
   a. Avocados
   b. Olives

List 6: Beverages, Snacks and Condiments

1. *Foods with Restrictions:*
   a. HIGH IN CALORIES: Frozen or canned fruit with sugar or honey added; jelly, jam, marmalade, honey; pure sugar candy such as gum drops, hard candy, mint patties (not chocolate); cakes, pies, cookies and puddings made with polyunsaturated fat in place of solid shortening; unsalted nuts, nonhydrogenated peanut butter; fruit drinks; sherbets; soda pop; wine, beer and whiskey (if allowed by physician).
   b. HIGH IN SODIUM: (Sodium restriction is necessary when the body holds rather than eliminates sodium and water.)

Salt, or sodium chloride ($NaCl$) is found in everything, but is most concentrated in certain foods that have been excluded from the food lists (such as bacon, ham, luncheon meat, potato chips, commercial pickles, ordinary canned soups). The greatest amount of sodium in the American diet comes from seasoning with table salt. Therefore, eliminating salt at the table and when possible, eliminating it in cooking, will greatly decrease the amount of sodium in your diet.

2. *Foods To Be Avoided:*
   a. Coconut and coconut oil
   b. Commercially fried foods such as potato chips and other deep fried snacks
   c. Whole milk puddings, chocolate pudding

Dietary control is your responsibility. However, it will be helpful for your family, especially the person who is actually preparing the food, to understand the diet as well. Arrangements will be made for you to see the hospital dietitian prior to discharge for additional instructions and possible questions.

GROUP C

For the first three months following valve replacement you should follow a low salt diet. Because this type of a diet has several modifications and variations, your doctor will request that a nutritionist talk with you to arrange the best possible diet plan.

V. INCISIONS (GROUPS B, C)

The chest incision is frequently quite sore and painful for several weeks following surgery. The breast bone (sternum) has been cut in half and then wired back together. The healing of the bone requires about six weeks, and until then the area may be tender and painful. If you wish, the doctor will provide pain medication to ease the problem when you are discharged.

Unless you have specific instructions to the contrary, you may bathe and shower, treating your incision as normal skin.

If you have a leg incision, you may find the following points helpful. These incisions often appear reddened from inflammation around the stitches. While this tends to subside with removal of the stitches, it may require additional time to disappear altogether. Swelling of the leg may occur as well. The best treatment for these problems is to elevate the leg while resting, apply warm (tap-water) compresses to the incision several times a day, and to wear an elastic stocking when up to reduce the swelling.

VI. MEDICATIONS (GROUPS A, B, C)

During the recovery phase following infarction or surgery, it is frequently necessary to use certain medications. Your doctors hope that this will be a

Figure 40   135

temporary need and they look forward to a time when no medicines will be necessary. Medications commonly used are:

1. Darvon (pink capsules)

   A drug used to relieve mild to moderate pain, in strength between aspirin and morphine. It may be habit-forming if used excessively.

2. Nitroglycerin (white tablets)

   These tablets are used under the tongue to relieve heart pain (angina).

3. Digoxin (white tablets)

   This is taken once a day to strengthen the heart beat and also to combat certain rhythm disturbances that occur following surgery.

4. Inderal (orange, green, yellow and other colors, round tablets, name and dose size on tablet)

   This drug is usually taken four times per day to reduce the heart rate. Through this and other actions, it reduces the work of the heart.

5. Warfarin (purple, orange, red and white tablets, size of dose on the tablet)

   This is a "blood thinner"—medical name, anticoagulant. This medicine is given once per day to slow down the clotting of blood. It is widely prescribed for people who have had blood vessel and heart surgery.

   Every patient with a new heart valve is advised to take warfarin for the first six weeks to three months following surgery. Then the doctor decides whether to continue the drug indefinitely, based on the patient's condition and the type of heart valve inserted.

VII. COMPLICATIONS

Now that you are about to go home the possibility of complications arising from your surgery progressively lessens. However, you should be aware of certain problems that might arise:

A. DEPRESSION

Some people experience a moderate depression or even severe mental depression following this surgery. This clears as they improve physically and lose the pain from the incision. This is a common event and only rarely develops into a serious problem.

B. INCISION HEALING PROBLEMS

Sometimes the incisions do not heal as intended because of infections or blood clots. Your doctor will outline home treatment methods to handle these problems if they occur. The incisions always heal with proper attention. Occasionally, infections or fluid collections occur on incisions weeks or even months after the surgery; these are always minor problems, but they are best handled by asking your doctor's advice.

C. PERICARDITIS

Sometimes the pericardium, a covering around the heart, becomes inflamed as a reaction to surgery. This usually is painful and causes prolonged chest pain following heart surgery. Treatment of pericarditis usually requires hospitalization and continued attention after discharge. It gradually subsides and does not mean that the operation has failed or that it will fail.

D. CHEST PAIN

In some cases the main purpose of the surgery is to eliminate or reduce anginal pain. If you have undergone surgery for this reason, and if you still feel some chest pain after surgery, it frequently is not true angina pain, but rather pain related to the healing surfaces inside the chest, or the bone itself. Sometimes it is difficult for the doctors to determine what is causing chest pain after the surgery, but in many cases we have seen that the pain is not true angina and that with time it does disappear.

Should real angina recur or be present following surgery, it can frequently be managed satisfactorily with medication.

Figure 41   137

Fig. 41.   Medical History Form

Name _____ Number _____ Date _____

Check X If Yes

PAST HISTORY		*FAMILY HISTORY*	
(Have you ever had?)		(Have any of your relatives had?)	
Rheumatic fever	( )	Heart attacks	( )
Heart murmur	( )	High blood pressure	( )
High blood pressure	( )	High cholesterol level	( )
Any heart trouble	( )	Diabetes	( )
Disease of arteries	( )	Congenital heart disease	( )
Varicose veins	( )	Heart operations	( )
Lung disease	( )	Other	( )
Operations	( )		
Injuries to back, etc.	( )		
Epilepsy	( )		

PRESENT SYMPTOMS REVIEW
(Have you recently had?)

Chest pain	( )	Coughing of blood	( )
Shortness of breath	( )	Back pain	( )
Heart palpitations	( )	Swollen, stiff or painful joints	( )
Cough on exertion	( )	Do you awaken at night to urinate? ( )	
Leg or ankle swelling	( )	Explain _____	

_____

RISK FACTORS

1. Smoking   Yes   No
   Do you smoke ( )   ( )
   Cigarettes   ( )   ( )   How many per day?__ How many years?__
   Cigar   ( )   ( )   How many per day?__ How many years?__
   Pipe   ( )   ( )   How many times a day?__ How many years?__
How old were you when you started? ____
In case you have stopped, when did you? _____
Why? _____

2. Diet
   What is your weight now?____ One year ago?____ At age 21?____
   Are you dieting?____ Why?_____

3. Exercise
   Do you engage in sports? ( )
   What? _____How often? ____
   How far do you think you walk each day? _____
   Is your occupation: Sedentary   ( )   Active ( )
                        Inactive   ( )   Heavy work ( )
   Do you have discomfort, shortness of breath or pain with moderate
   exercise? ( )
   Specify _____
   Were you a high school or college athlete? ( ) Specify _____

Fig. 42. Informed Consent Form

I desire to engage voluntarily in the Cardiac Rehabilitation Program in order to improve my physical fitness. My participation in this program has been recommended and approved by my physician, Dr. _____ of _____ clinic.

Before I enter the exercise phase of the program, I will have a clinical evaluation. This evaluation will include a medical history and physical examination consisting of, but not limited to, measurements of heart rate and blood pressure, ECG at rest and during exercise. The exercise test that I will undergo will be performed on a treadmill, with the amount of effort increasing gradually. This increase in effort will continue until a predetermined heart rate response is achieved, or other symptoms such as fatigue, shortness of breath, or chest pain may appear, which would indicate to me to stop. During the performance of the test, a physician and trained observers will keep under surveillance my pulse, blood pressure and electrocardiogram. Oxygen intake may also be measured. There exists the possibility of certain changes occurring during the exercise test. They include abnormal blood pressure, pulse rate, and very rare instances of "heart attack." Every effort will be made to minimize the possibility of such undesirable changes by an entrance interview, and by observations made during testing. Emergency equipment is available to deal with unusual situations that may arise. The purpose of this evaluation is twofold: (1) to detect any condition that would indicate that I should not engage in this exercise program; (2) to determine the level of exercise for me during the three-per-week exercise sessions.

The exercise sessions that I will become involved in will follow personalized exercise levels based upon the laboratory evaluation, and will be carefully regulated by the supervisor of the exercise program. The amount of exercise will be regulated on the basis of my exercise tolerance. The exercise activities are designed to place a gradually increasing work load on the circulation system (cardiovascular system), and thereby to improve its function. The reaction of the cardiovascular system to such activities cannot always be predicted with complete accuracy. Therefore, there is the risk of certain changes occurring during or following the exercise. These changes include abnormalities of blood pressure or heart rate, or ineffective "heart function," and in rare, instances "heart attacks" or "cardiac arrest."

Before initially participating in the exercise phase of the Cardiac Rehabilitation Program, I will be instructed regarding the signs and symptoms that I should report promptly to the supervisor of the exercises and that will alert me to modify my activities. I also will be observed by the supervisor of the exercises, or an assigned assistant, who will be alert to changes that would suggest that I modify my exercise. Every effort will be made to avoid such events by the entrance interview, the preliminary medical examination (laboratory evaluation), and by the observations made during the exercise sessions. Emergency equipment and trained personnel are available to deal with and minimize the dangers of untoward events should they occur.

The information that is obtained during the laboratory evaluations and exercise sessions of the Cardiac Rehabilitation Program will be treated as privileged and confidential, and will not be released or revealed to any nonmedical person without my expressed written consent. The information obtained, however, may be used for a statistical or scientific purpose with my right of privacy retained. I also approve of periodic forwarding to my physician of data relative to the laboratory evaluation(s) and my involvement in the exercise sessions.

I have read the foregoing and I understand it. Any questions that have arisen or occurred to me have been answered to my satisfaction.

Signed:

_____
Patient

_____
Date

_____
Physician

_____
Program Director

_____
Witness

_____
Date

Fig. 43.   Pre GXT Data Form

Name: _____ Age: _____ Date: _____
Attending Physician: _____ Eval. No. 1__ 2__ 3__ 4__
Height: _____ ft. _____ inches_____cm   Weight: _____ lbs. _____kg.
Resting HR _____ Resting BP __/__ Resting (Supine) ECG _____

Anthropometric Studies

Measurement	Value	Conversion Value
Constant	8.987	A. _____
Weight	_____Kg-lbs	B. _____
Wrist diameter	_____cm	C. _____
Forearm Circumference	_____cm	D. _____
Add: A + B + C + D		E. _____
Max. Abdominal Circum.	_____cm	F. _____
Hip Circumference	_____cm	G. _____
		H. _____

Subtract H from E—This gives the LBW (Lead Body Weight) in kg.

RESPIRATORY STUDIES
Vital capacity: Pr _____   Ob _____   % _____
Forced expiratory
    volume, 1 sec.:   Pr _____   Ob _____   % _____
Midexpiratory Flow Rate   Ob _____   L/min.

BLOOD ANALYSIS

Hematocrit	_____%	*MEDICATION:*
Hemoglobin	_____Hb/100 ml	
Cholesterol #1	_____mg %	
Cholesterol #2	_____mg %	
Lactic acid (Resting)	_____mg/ml	
Lactic Acid (Exercise)	_____mg/ml	
ECG Studies (check)		
Supine	_____	Posthyperventilation _____
Standing	_____	

Figure 44   141

Fig. 44.   Graded Exercise Test Form

GRADED EXERCISE   Name: _____

I. Preliminary Data

Cardiac Patient___ Prone Patient___ Predicted Maximum___ ___% Max.___

II. Graded Exercise Test

  A. Exercise Phase

     Phase   BP   HR (B/min)   VO$_2$ (ml/kg/min)

    (a) 1.5 mph-.0% Grade

         :45-1:00 minute   ___/___ _____ _____

        2:45-3:00 minutes   ___/___ _____ _____

    (b) 2.0 mph-.0% Grade

        3:45-4:00 minutes   ___/___ _____ _____

        5:45-6:00 minutes   ___/___ _____ _____

    (c) 2.5 mph-.0% Grade

        6:45-7:00 minutes   ___/___ _____ _____

        8:45-9:00 minutes   ___/___ _____ _____

    (d) 3.0 mph-.0% Grade

        9:45-10:00 minutes   ___/___ _____ _____

      11:45-12:00 minutes   ___/___ _____ _____

    (e) 3.0 mph-5% Grade

      12:45-13:00 minutes   ___/___ _____ _____

      14:45-15:00 minutes   ___/___ _____ _____

    (f) 3.0 mph-7½% Grade

      15:45-16:00 minutes   ___/___ _____ _____

      17:45-18:00 minutes   ___/___ _____ _____

    (g) 3.0 mph-10% Grade

      18:45-19:00 minutes   ___/___ _____ _____

      20:45-21:00 minutes   ___/___ _____ _____

  Maximal Values   ___/___ _____ _____

  B. Recovery Phase

            BP   HR (B/min)   BP   HR (B/min)

    2:00 ___/___ _____   8:00 ___/___ _____

    4:00 ___/___ _____   10:00 ___/___ _____

    6:00 ___/___ _____

Fig. 45.   Dietary Information Form

Name _____Date _____

A diet, tailored to individual needs by a nutritionist, seems desirable for many participants in conjunction with the normal activities of the Cardiac Rehabilitation Program. Please complete the following:

1. How much exercise do you receive in a normal day, other than through the Cardiac Rehabilitation Program? _____

2. What is your occupation? _____

3. What medication(s) are you presently taking? _____
   _____
   _____

4. Are you presently on a diet? ____ If so, has the diet been suggested by your physician? ____ Describe the diet: _____
   _____

5. Where are your meals eaten? _____

6. Who prepares your meals? _____

7. How often do you eat in restaurants? _____

8. Does your eating pattern vary on weekends? _____
   _____
   _____

"NORMAL" 24 HOUR *EAT* AND *DRINK* HABITS

Indicate below the food and drink you normally consume daily. It is extremely important that you be honest regarding what you eat and drink during a 24-hour period.

| *BREAKFAST* | *NOON MEAL* | *EVENING MEAL* |

| *Snack* | *Snack* | *Snack* |

9. Do you consume alcohol on a regular basis? ____ If so, in what form is the drink? _____ How much would you consume in an average day? _____ In the above 24-hour period, was anything omitted that normally would not have been? _____ Explain: _____
   _____
   _____

10. Do you take any protein, vitamin or mineral supplements? _____
    Amount _____ Kind _____

Figure 46   143

Fig. 46.   Consent to Take and Use Pictures Form

DATE: _____

I am a participant in the Cardiac Rehabilitation Program and understand that pictures of program participants for use in educational materials, studies, reports and books will be periodically taken on an unannounced basis. I request and consent to the taking of pictures of me participating in the program and request and consent to the use of the pictures in educational materials, studies, reports and books. I understand that pictures may be used in publications with national distribution and slides, etc., may be shown at national conventions with large audiences.

Signed: _____

Print Name _____

Fig. 47.   Purposes of the Graded Exercise Test

I. DIAGNOSTIC GRADED EXERCISE TEST (DGXT)

  A. Purpose—Diagnosis of the presence of coronary artery disease.
  B. Degree of effort—Symptom-limited maximal or maximal.

II. NONDIAGNOSTIC (FUNCTIONAL) GRADED EXERCISE TEST (FGXT)

  A. Types
     1. Sports medicine FGXT.
     2. Prevention, intervention, rehabilitation FGXT.

  B. Purpose
     1. Sports medicine FGXT
        a. Research.
        b. Development of training and conditioning program.
     2. Prevention, intervention, rehabilitation FGXT
        a. Exercise prescription.
        b. Therapeutic evaluation.
        c. Determination of physiologic effect of exercise involvement.
        d. Motivation.

  C. Degree of effort
     1. Sports medicine FGXT: Maximal.
     2. Prevention, intervention FGXT: Symptom-limited maximal or maximal.
     3. Rehabilitation FGXT:
        a. Hospital discharge FGXT: Symptom-limited or submaximal.
        b. Phase II, Phase III, and Repeat FGXTs: Symptom-limited maximal or maximal.

Figure 48   145

Fig. 48.   Cooper Heart Rate Prediction Table*

AGE	V. P. & POOR	FAIR	GOOD	AGE	V. P. & POOR	FAIR	GOOD
20	201	201	196	45	174	183	183
21	199	200	196	46	173	182	183
22	198	199	195	47	172	181	182
23	197	198	195	48	171	181	182
24	196	198	194	49	170	180	181
25	195	197	194	50	168	179	180
26	194	196	193	51	167	179	180
27	193	196	193	52	166	178	179
28	192	195	192	53	165	177	179
29	191	193	192	54	164	176	178
30	190	193	191	55	163	176	178
31	189	193	191	56	162	175	177
32	188	192	190	57	161	174	177
33	187	191	189	58	160	174	176
34	186	191	189	59	159	173	176
35	184	190	188	60	158	172	175
36	183	189	188	61	157	172	175
37	182	189	187	62	156	171	174
38	181	188	187	63	155	170	174
39	180	187	186	64	154	169	173
40	179	186	186	65	152	169	173
41	178	186	185	66	151	168	172
42	177	185	185	67	150	167	171
43	176	184	184	68	149	167	171
44	175	184	184	69	148	166	170
				70	147	165	170

Date: _____

Category: _____

Percentage: _____

*Used with the permission of Kenneth Cooper, M.D., Cooper Clinic, Dallas Texas.

Fig. 49.   GXT Summary Form

GUNDERSEN CLINIC, LTD.   DATE: _____
GXT REPORT

Patient: _____ Physician: _____

Clinic No: _____ Cardiologist: _____

Patient Ht: _____cm.   Wgt: _____kg.   Age: _____ yrs.

Resting (Supine) HR: _____   BP:_____

Predicted Max HR: _____   90% _____   70% _____

Predicted Max BP: Systolic _____   Diastolic _____

Attained Max HR _____   SBP _____   DBP_____

Predicted RPP Max _____ Attained RPP Max _____

Predicted VO$_2$ Max_____ L/min _____ml/kg/min

Attained VO$_2$ _____L/min _____ml/kg/min

Functional Aerobic Impairment (FAI):_____

FAI (   ) + Att. VO$_2$ (   ) = 100% VO$_2$ Max (Bruce nomogram)

Energy Expenditure (   ) K.Cal   (   ) METS

Functional Class (AHA): (_____) Fitness Level (_____)

Reason for Stopping: _____

Resting (standing) ECG _____

Post Hypervent. ECG _____

1. EXERCISE ECG:

2. POST EXERCISE ECG:

3. CONCLUSION:

GC 1317 475

Figure 49   147

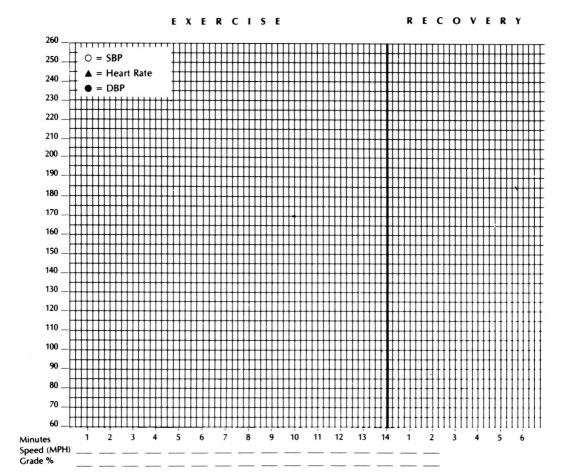

Signature: _____

Fig. 50.   Functional GXT Termination Points

Patient Classification	Evaluation No.	%	Cooper Category*
Cardiac Patient	1	65	Poor
	2	75	Fair
	3	85	Good
(and all future FGXTs)			
Cardiac-Prone Patient	1	85	Poor
	2	85	Fair
	3	85	Good
(and all future FGXTs)			

*See Figure 48.

Figure 51   149

Fig. 51.   Treadmill Protocols (Functional GXT, Beginning and Advanced)

Wilson Beginning Functional Graded Exercise Test (B-FGXT)

					Mets*	
Time	Speed	Grade (%)	VO$_2$ ml/kg/min	actual	approximate	increase
3	1.5	0	4.90	1.40	1.5	
6	2.0	0	6.90	1.98	2.0	.5
9	2.5	0	8.68	2.48	2.5	.5
12	3.0	0	10.42	2.97	3.0	.5
15	3.0	5	17.55	5.02	5.0	2.0
18	3.0	7.5	21.12	6.04	6.0	1.0
21	3.0	10	24.69	7.05	7.0	1.0

Wilson Advanced Functional Graded Exercise Test (A-FGXT)

					Mets*	
Time	Speed	Grade %	VO$_2$ ml/kg/min	actual	approximate	increase
3	1.5	10	12.30	3.50	3.5	
6	2.0	12.5	18.84	5.38	5.5	2.0
9	2.5	15	26.52	7.50	7.5	2.0
12	3.0	15	31.83	9.09	9.0	1.5
15	3.5	15	37.13	10.61	10.5	1.5
18	4.0	15	42.44	12.12	12.0	1.5
21	4.5	15	47.75	13.64	13.5	1.5

*1 met = 3.5 ml/kg/min

Fig. 52.   ECG-GXT Recording Procedures

1. Prior to DGXT (supine, standing, posthyperventilation)
2. During DGXT
   a. Periodic during, 2 or 3 minute (exercise set, 3-lead)
   b. Maximal exercise (12-lead)
   c. Immediate postexercise (12-lead), within 20 seconds
3. Recovery (2 to 3 minutes, 12-lead)

Figure 53   151

Fig. 53.   First Laboratory Evaluation Physician Memo

TO: Primary Physician
FROM: Program Director
RE: Laboratory Evaluation Flow Sheet

Enclosed is a copy of the Laboratory Evaluation Flow Sheet for ____
_____. Please feel free
to contact me if you would like a copy of the resting, exercise (GXT), or
recovery electrocardiograms relative to your patient's Laboratory Evaluation. Upon administration of each subsequent Laboratory Evaluation of
your patient, you will receive a revised Laboratory Evaluation Flow Sheet.

In addition to the Laboratory Evaluation Flow Sheet, you will receive
monthly an Exercise Session Flow Sheet regarding your patient. The
exercise Progress Report Flow Sheet will inform you of the patient's weight,
percentage of attendance, exercise heart rate, and exercise tolerance during
the most recent month, as well as compare it to the entire period in which the
patient has been a participant in the Cardiac Rehabilitation Program.

Please feel free to contact me if you have any questions concerning
either of the described flow sheets. Your cooperation concerning the Cardiac
Rehabilitation Program is sincerely appreciated.

Date: _____

Fig. 54.   Subsequent Laboratory Evaluation Physician Memo

TO: Primary Physician
FROM: Program Director
RE: Laboratory Evaluation Flow Sheet

    Enclosed is a copy of the revised Laboratory Evaluation Flow Sheet for _____. The patient recently received his/her _____ Laboratory Evaluation, and data relative to such is entered on the flow sheet. Upon administration of each subsequent Laboratory Evaluation, you will receive a revised Laboratory Evaluation Flow Sheet.

    Please feel free to contact me if you have any questions concerning the enclosed flow sheet. Also, feel free to contact me if you would like a copy of the resting, exercise (GXT), or recovery electrocardiogram relative to your patient's most recent Laboratory Evaluation.

    Thank you for your cooperation concerning the Cardiac Rehabilitation Program.

Date: _____

Figure 55   153

Fig. 55. Laboratory Evaluation Flow Sheet, Physician

Patient's Name _____
Clinic No. _____
Referring Physician
_____
Attending Physician
_____

Side 1

DATE									
PATIENT STATUS: Cardiac Prone (CP) Diagnostic (D) Post Infarct (PI), mths. Post Surgery (PS), mths. Rehab. Status (RS), mths.									

RESTING DATA

HR (Beats/min.)									
Blood Pressure									

ANTHROPOMETRIC DATA

Weight (lb/kg)									
Body Fat Behnke (%) / Lange (%)									

PULMONARY DATA

Vital Capacity (L)									
Forced Expiratory Volume (L)									
Mid Flow (L/Min.)									

BLOOD ANALYSIS DATA

Hematocrit (%)									
Hemoglobin (Hb/100 ml)									
Cholesterol (mg%)									
Lactic Acid (mg/ml) (resting)									
Lactic Acid (mg/ml) (exercise)									

Fig. 55 (Continued)

Side 2   Name _____

DATE OF TEST											
Minutes of Exercise Completed											
Speed and Grade At Which Exercise Was Completed											
Maximum Blood Pressure Achieved During Exercise											
HR "Cut Off" Point / Predicted Max. HR = %											
Maximum Heart Rate Achieved During Exercise											
Rate—Mean Blood Pressure Product											
VO_2 Achieved / VO_2 Calculated = %											
Maximum k cal/min Utilized											
Minutes After Exercise for Blood Pressure to Return to Baseline											
Minutes After Exercise for Heart Rate to Return to Baseline											
Reason for Stopping Test											
Positive (+) or Negative (−) GXT											

Figure 56   155

Fig. 56.   Laboratory Evaluation Parameter Explanation, Patient

The parameters discussed below are those that are measured during the laboratory evaluations of participants in the Cardiac Rehabilitation Program. This information is provided to inform you of what is being done in these laboratory evaluations, and is not necessarily a complete medical explanation of each parameter. The effect of exercise on each parameter is also included. The lack of a desirable effect of exercise on a parameter does not necessarily indicate development of a medical condition that would warrant your concern. Such an interpretation should be left to your referring physician, who receives a copy of this data after each laboratory evaluation.

PRELIMINARY DATA

Heart rate is defined as the number of times that the heart contracts or beats during a one-minute period. Exercise increases the efficiency of one's musculature, with the result that less blood flow to the muscles will be required each minute for a given level of exercise. Accordingly, after exercise training the heart rate may decrease.

Blood pressure is the pressure, measured in millimeters of mercury, at which the blood passes through the vessels. Exercise is thought to enable arteries to remain more distensible, prevent build-up of deposits in artery walls, reduce nervous tension which blocks blood flow, and increase the number of capillaries in the tissue area. All of these factors may lead to a general lowering of blood pressure with exercise.

Weight and fat percentage may both decrease with exercise. If the participant's caloric intake remains constant and his caloric expenditure is increased through exercise, the net result should be a loss of weight and a decrease in fat percentage.

BLOOD ANALYSIS DATA

Cholesterol is a lipid that is secreted by the liver in stressful situations to act as a reserve source of fuel. An excess of cholesterol in the blood is thought to result in the formation of deposits on artery walls, thus decreasing blood flow. Exercise utilizes the cholesterol as a fuel source. Nervous tension is also a stress that causes the liver to secrete cholesterol. Exercise is thought to reduce these tensions and thus can cause a decrease in the cholesterol level in the blood.

GRADED EXERCISE TEST (GXT) DATA

Heart Rate Cut-off is the maximal heart rate that a participant will be exercised to during his Graded Exercise Test. This cut-off point has been predetermined on the basis of age and medical status of the patient.

Maximal Blood Pressure is the highest pressure reached during exercise. Exercise blood pressure should decrease, for the same reason that resting blood pressure decreases, with participation in regular exercise sessions.

Minutes Completed is the amount of time that a person was on the treadmill or bicycle until his heart rate reached the cut-off point or he discontinued for some other reason. With exercise, the minutes completed should increase from laboratory evaluation to laboratory evaluation.

RECOVERY GRADED EXERCISE TEST (GXT) DATA

Recovery (postexercise) measures should show a decrease as the result of regular exercise. Exercise will better enable the cardiovascular system to carry oxygen to the fatigued tissues and to carry waste products from these tissues in greater amounts and at a faster rate. The faster the tissues are brought to their resting condition, the faster one will recover to his resting heart rate and blood pressure. Therefore, the recovery (postexercise) heart rate and blood pressure approach resting values (pre-exercise) faster in the conditioned individual than the nonconditioned individual.

Figure 57   157

Fig. 57.   First Laboratory Evaluation Patient Memo

TO: Patient

FROM: Program Director

Enclosed is a summary of the data collected during your entrance laboratory evaluation to the Cardiac Rehabilitation Program. Also enclosed is an
explanation of the data collected during the laboratory evaluation.

If you have any questions concerning the enclosed, feel free to contact
me at your convenience.

We are happy to have you with us.

Fig. 58.   Subsequent Laboratory Evaluation Patient Memo

TO: Patient

FROM: Program Director

Enclosed is a summary of the data collected during your recent laboratory evaluation and a comparison of the data to the data collected during your
_____ evaluation. The summary sheet also includes a comparison of
your exercise tolerance and exercise heart rate from the time you entered the
program until the present. If you have any questions concerning the enclosed
material, feel free to contact me at your convenience.

I hope you are enjoying the Cardiac Rehabilitation Program and feel that
you are benefiting physiologically.

Figure 59   159

Fig. 59. Laboratory Evaluation Flow Sheet, Patient

	__/__/__ Date	__/__/__ Date	__/__/__ Date
Resting Data			
−HR (beats/min)	_____	_____	_____
−SBP/DBP (Syst.-Diast.)	_____	_____	_____
Anthropometric Data			
−Weight (lb/kg)	___/___	___/___	___/___
−Body Fat % (Behnke)	_____	_____	_____
−Body Fat % (Lange Caliper)	_____	_____	_____
Blood Analysis Data			
−Cholesterol (mg %)	_____	_____	_____
Exercise Data			
Heart Rate Cut-Off Point (beats/min)	_____	_____	_____
−Maximal SBP/DBP	___/___	___/___	___/___
+Minutes Completed	_____	_____	_____
Postexercise Recovery Data			
SBP/DBP (Syst.-Diast.)			
−2:00 min.	_____	_____	_____
−6:00 min.	_____	_____	_____
Heart Rate			
−2:00 min.	_____	_____	_____
−6:00 min.	_____	_____	_____
+*Current Exercise Tolerance*	_____	_____	_____

+These values should increase with an increase in cardiovascular endurance.

−These values should decrease with an increase in cardiovascular endurance.

Fig. 60.   Exercise Prescription Form

Patient's Name _____

Date	GXT Max. Target	Previous Exercise Sessions, Target HR	Future Exercise Sessions, Target HR	Prescriber
____	_____	_____	_____	_____
____	_____	_____	_____	_____
____	_____	_____	_____	_____
____	_____	_____	_____	_____
____	_____	_____	_____	_____
____	_____	_____	_____	_____
____	_____	_____	_____	_____
____	_____	_____	_____	_____
____	_____	_____	_____	_____
____	_____	_____	_____	_____
____	_____	_____	_____	_____

Figure 61   161

Fig. 61.   Patient Orientation to Pool Phase

INTRODUCTION

We welcome you as a participant in the Cardiac Rehabilitation Program. The following is important information we wish you to understand prior to entering the pool phase of the program.

POOL INFORMATION

1. Equipment—bring a comfortable swimsuit, towels, bathing cap for women and shower items (soap, soap dish, shampoo, etc.).
2. First day in the pool—meet in the Human Performance Laboratory (where you had your laboratory evaluation).
3. Women will be issued a lock and locker to use on a permanent basis.
4. Men will bring their *own* locks to be used on issued lockers. Combination locks are recommended.
5. Always keep your lockers locked. There have been a few cases of vandalism.

POOL PROCEDURES AND TIME SCHEDULE

Before 5:00   Before entering pool area, weigh yourself in the locker room and remember what your weight is.

5:00   As you enter the pool area, use one of the big clocks to time your entering resting heart rate for ten seconds. To save time and to be more efficient, remember your weight and entering heart rate. Give your last name, weight and heart rate to the recorder. (Example: Jones, 120 lbs., 15)

5:00–5:10   1. Warm-up phase. Spread out standing on the exercise mats with your back to the wall. Warm-up exercises will be done for two five-minute intervals.
              2. All warm-up exercises are performed to a four-count rhythm. Because you are a new member to the program, for the first three weeks you are to follow the schedule below in performing your warm-up exercises:
                 a. first exercise session: 1 of each exercise
                 b. sessions 2, 3, and 4:   4 repetitions of each exercise
                 c. sessions 5, 6, 7, 8, 9: 6 repetitions of each exercise
                 d. remaining sessions   8 repetitions of each exercise
              3. After the first five minutes of exercise, take pulse for ten seconds, yell out last name and pulse to the recorder (you will be instructed to do this by your Exercise Leader). After the second five-minute interval of exercise, take another pulse and yell out last name and pulse to the recorder.

Note: No two people are alike; consequently, your pulse rate prescription relates only to your condition. It is imperative that you follow the foregoing schedule only if you are "feeling good," have no adverse effects from the exercise (muscle and/or joint soreness), and are not experiencing unusual cardiac symptoms.

4. Once you start the fourth warm-up exercises and if you are beyond the ninth session (fourth week), do not become motionless between individual exercises, even while you are taking your pulse or waiting to get into the pool. Always keep your legs moving by "walking in place" if you are standing up, or by bending your knees if you are sitting down.

5:10–5:15 Warm-up exercises in the pool
1. You will do water exercises to adjust your body to the water temperature of the pool.
2. After the water exercises, you will take your pulse and have it recorded.

5:15–5:30 Walking and swimming
1. Everyone is given a prescribed heart rate. Make sure you know what your prescribed heart rate is. This heart rate tells us at which level you can safely exercise. It is not necessary to obtain that particular heart rate; however, it is important to try to stay within two heart beats *below* your prescribed heart rate. For instance, if your prescribed heart rate is 20, try to stay around 18 or below. You should never go above your exercise prescription.
2. To begin with, walk at a comfortable pace from width to width:
Example:

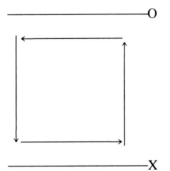

walk from X-O, back O-X, this is considered two widths.

a. Initially, walk two widths for the first couple of days until you feel comfortable and adjusted to the pro-

Figure 61   163

gram. Eventually you will gradually increase the number of widths. The exercise leader will notify you of the progression to follow.

b. After two widths, take pulse, raise two fingers in the air to get recorder's attention, shout last name, pulse rate, number of widths (for example: Jones, 16 for 2).

Thereafter, after two widths, take pulse. Remember, a lot depends on how you personally feel and how your heart reacts to exercise. There is no set progression because everyone works in different stages.

c. Depending on the individual's progression, you will learn to swim the elementary back stroke. We have qualified instructors to teach you how to swim.

d. After three months you will be re-evaluated to determine whether you should proceed to the track phase of the program.

5:50–6:00   Cool-down exercises—everyone comes to the shallow end of the pool with the exercise leader for some cool-down exercises. Upon completion of the cool-down exercises, take five consecutive heart rates and have heart rates recorded.

IMPORTANT INFORMATION

1. Prior to coming to the exercise sessions:

Do not eat or drink (water is permitted) at least three hours prior to entering the exercise program.

If you experience any *unaccustomed symptoms of pain, discomfort or soreness,* let the staff know *before* you start exercising. Also, while exercising, if you notice any unaccustomed symptoms, slow down and inform one of the staff members.

Always report any unaccustomed symptoms, whether of joint, muscular, or cardiac nature. The most important factor in regulating your exercise level is how you feel. If you are "feeling good" during the exercise session, you should attempt to reach your maximum allowable heart rate. If you are not feeling good, you should (1) let the Exercise Leader in charge know, and (2) take it easy during the exercise session (do not attempt to reach your prescribed heart rate).

2. Be prompt; the session lasts from 5:00 to 6:00. No leaving early; inform staff if early dismissal is necessary.

3. Pulse taking. You have been instructed on how to take your pulse. Practice taking your pulse. Try using both methods, at your wrist and

your neck. While in our program, if you have a difficult time taking your pulse, request assistance from your exercise assistant or the supervising staff member.

4. Heart rate control. ALWAYS know your maximum allowable heart rate. The Exercise Leader in charge will know this value. When you take your heart rate, take it *immediately* as you come off of your last walking step. Be accurate in taking your heart rate. Always count the first beat as zero, then, one, two, three. . . .

5. Bring robe, towel, and slippers with you to the pool area.

6. While exercising, breathe normally and naturally.

7. *Do not*
   a. Hold your breath, even for an instant.
   b. Swim under water.
   c. Dive or jump into the water.

8. Always do the warm-up and cool-down exercises.

9. Be accurate in reporting your distance (laps) to heart rate recorders.

10. Take a medium warm shower after the exercise session. Do not take a cold or hot shower.

11. Upon leaving the locker room at the end of the day, be sure to dress appropriately and have your hair dry, especially during the cold weather.

12. If planning to miss an exercise session, please notify the staff by calling the Cardiac Rehabilitation Office and report your absence.

13. Don't forget your belongings when you leave. Men are required to take their locks home with them.

14. Keep all insurance forms up to date.

Figure 62   165

Fig. 62.   Patient Orientation to Track Phase

INTRODUCTION

You are now ready to enter the track phase of the Cardiac Rehabilitation Program. The track phase will have many similarities to the pool phase which you just completed; however, it is important that you realize that the track phase is a lot more strenuous and demanding on the heart. For this reason, it is extremely important that you understand these instructions and ask questions when in doubt.

TRACK INFORMATION
1. Equipment:

Shoes. Wear low-cut running shoes with arch supports and at least one-half-inch thick soles. We suggest that you not wear flat rubber-sole basketball-type shoes, but purchase a good pair of running shoes.

Socks. Socks should always be worn while walking or jogging. Any comfortable all-cotton brand will be adequate.

Shirts and Pants. Cardiac Program shirts and running shorts can be obtained from the Exercise Leader in charge of the track. There is a charge for this apparel and you will be billed by mail.
2. The track measures ⅛ of a mile; thus, eight laps on the inside lane equals one mile.
3. You will notice cardiac patients who exercise on their own. This is the Advanced Group. You will *not* exercise on your own until you have satisfactorily completed a Graded Exercise Test that indicates you are ready to enter the advanced phase and you are given the "go-ahead" from the Executive Director of the Cardiac Rehabilitation Program. You will be given this Graded Exercise Test to enter the Advanced Group after spending three months on the track phase.

TRACK PROCEDURES AND TIME SCHEDULE

Before 5:00   Weigh yourself in the locker room.
5:00   Upon arriving at the track area, take a resting pulse for ten seconds. To save time and to be more efficient, remember your weight and your entering heart rate. Give your last name, weight and heart rate to the recorder. (Example: Jones, 120 lbs., 15)
5:00–5:10   1. Warm-up phase. Spread out and be prepared for the warm-up exercises to be led by the Exercise Leader.
              2. All warm-up exercises are performed to a four-count rhythm. Because you are a new member on the track, for

the first two weeks you are to follow the schedule below
in performing your warm-up exercises:

a. Sessions 1, 2, and 3   4 repetitions of each exercise
b. Sessions 4, 5, and 6   6 repetitions of each exercise
c. Remaining sessions   8 repetitions of each exercise

3. After five minutes of warm-up, take pulse for ten seconds, yell out last name and heart rate to recorder. After
   the second five-minute interval of exercise, take another
   pulse and yell out your last name and heart rate to recorder.

   Note: No two people are alike; consequently, your heart
   rate prescription relates only to your condition. It is
   imperative that you follow the foregoing schedule only if
   you are "feeling good," have no adverse effects from the
   exercise (muscle and/or joint soreness), and have no
   unaccustomed cardiac symptoms.

4. At the end of warm-up exercises, patients will walk one-
   half lap utilizing long strides to stretch. Arm exercises
   are also done. This will be performed with the Exercise
   Leader.

5:10–5:40   Walking and jogging, depending on individual prescriptions. After your one-half lap of long strides, you will be
ready to start your running prescription. You should
follow the below indicated schedule on running.

1. Sessions 1, 2, 3 on track: The participant should only
   walk during the first three sessions. Walk at a pace that
   will elicit a heart rate within two beats below your allowable heart rate. Take and report your heart rate to the
   recorder after each two laps of walking.

2. Sessions 4, 5, 6: Jog only on "straight-aways." Stay in
   one of the outside three lanes. Take and report your heart
   rate to the recorder after each two laps.

3. Sessions 7, 8, 9: Jog one lap at a time and take and report
   heart rate. If, by session 9, your heart rate has been under
   your maximum allowed heart rate, jog two laps before
   taking heart rate.

4. Remaining sessions: Begin the first few sessions by jogging two laps before taking heart rate. The distance can
   then be increased, depending on the response of your
   heart rate and the occurrence of any symptoms that may
   curtail either the speed or distance you jog.

5:40–5:55   Continue running prescription. Upon completion of your
running prescription, if time permits, you can either walk
slow laps or play volleyball. If you decide to play volleyball,
remember, keep it low-keyed—do not get too competitive.

Figure 62   167

5:55–6:00   Cool-down exercises, very similar to cool-down period in swimming phase. You will gather together with the Exercise Leader, do some cool-down exercises, and then take five consecutive heart rates and have these recorded.

IMPORTANT INFORMATION

1. Prior to coming to the exercise sessions:

   Do not eat or drink (water is permitted) at least three hours prior to entering the exercise program.

   If you experience any *unaccustomed symptoms of pain, discomfort or soreness,* let the staff know *before* you start exercising. Also, while exercising, if you notice any unaccustomed symptoms, slow down and inform one of the staff members.

   Always report any unaccustomed symptoms, whether of joint, muscular, or cardiac nature. The most important factor in regulating your exercise level is how you feel. If you are "feeling good" during the exercise session, you should attempt to reach your maximum allowable heart rate. If you are not feeling good, you should (1) let the Exercise Leaders in charge know, and (2) take it easy during the exercise session (do not attempt to reach your prescribed heart rate).

2. Be prompt; the session lasts from 5:00 to 6:00. No leaving early; inform staff if early dismissal is necessary.

3. Heart rate control. ALWAYS know your maximum allowable heart rate. The Exercise Leader in charge will know this value. When you take your heart rate, take it *immediately* as you come off of your last walking or jogging step. Be accurate in taking your heart rate. Always count the first beat as zero, then one, two, three. . . .

4. Running style. The jog should be relaxed and your breathing should be easy and with a rhythm. Use your arms and do not clinch your fists. Do not sprint or run on toes.

5. If you get "shin splints" from either walking or jogging, let the Exercise Leader in charge know. Shin splints are aching pains that radiate down the front of the shin or sometimes in the back. They can be alleviated and in most cases prevented by placing the feet about hip-width apart and leaning against a wall. The feet should remain flat on the floor and the back kept straight.

6. If you walk because you cannot jog, be sure to walk at a fast enough pace that will elicit a heart rate approaching your maximum allowable heart rate.

7. Do not perform any breath-holding or isometric-type exercises while exercising and running; breathe normally and naturally.

8. Always do the warm-up and cool-down exercises.

9. Be accurate in reporting your distances (laps) to heart rate recorders.

10. Take a medium-warm shower after the exercise session. Do not take a cold or hot shower.
11. Upon leaving the locker room at the end of the day, be sure that you dress appropriately and your hair is dry.
12. If planning to miss any exercise sessions, please notify the staff of your planned absence.
13. Don't forget your belongings.
14. Keep all insurance forms up-to-date.

Figure 63   169

Fig. 63.   Exercise Therapy Session Daily Data Sheet*

	Patient
NAME _____	Pool/Track/Adv./Beg. No. _____

Date _____, Weight _____, Ent. HR _____

Maximum Prescribed HR ☐

Warm-up Phase HR (1) _____, (2) _____
EXERCISE:

HR	D	HR	D	HR	D	HR	D	HR	D

TOTAL _____ POST EX. HR (1)_____,
(2)_____, (3)_____ (4)_____ (5)_____.

Date _____, Weight _____, Ent. HR _____

Maximum Prescribed HR ☐

Warm-up Phase HR (1) _____, (2) _____
EXERCISE:

HR	D	HR	D	HR	D	HR	D	HR	D

TOTAL _____ POST EX. HR (1)_____,
(2)_____, (3)_____ (4)_____ (5)_____.

Date _____, Weight _____, Ent. HR _____

Maximum Prescribed HR ☐

Warm-up Phase HR (1) _____, (2) _____
EXERCISE:

HR	D	HR	D	HR	D	HR	D	HR	D

TOTAL _____ POST EX. HR (1)_____,
(2)_____, (3)_____ (4)_____ (5)_____.

Date _____, Weight _____, Ent. HR _____

Maximum Prescribed HR ☐

Warm-up Phase HR (1) _____, (2) _____
EXERCISE:

HR	D	HR	D	HR	D	HR	D	HR	D

TOTAL _____ POST EX. HR (1)_____,
(2)_____, (3)_____ (4)_____ (5)_____.

Date _____, Weight _____, Ent. HR _____

Maximum Prescribed HR ☐

Warm-up Phase HR (1) _____, (2) _____
EXERCISE:

HR	D	HR	D	HR	D	HR	D	HR	D

TOTAL _____ POST EX. HR (1)_____,
(2)_____, (3)_____ (4)_____ (5)_____.

Date _____, Weight _____, Ent. HR _____

Maximum Prescribed HR ☐

Warm-up Phase HR (1) _____, (2) _____
EXERCISE:

HR	D	HR	D	HR	D	HR	D	HR	D

TOTAL _____ POST EX. HR (1)_____,
(2)_____, (3)_____ (4)_____ (5)_____.

---

*HR = Heart rate.

Fig. 64.   Transfer Letter, Physician

TO: Primary Physician
FROM: Program Director

We are writing concerning the transfer of your patient _____ to
the Advanced Group of the Cardiac Rehabilitation Program. The Advanced
Cardiac Group, which meets twice a week (Tuesday-Thursday) for
nonphysician-supervised exercise sessions, is available to (1) those who are
prone to coronary heart disease and have demonstrated a moderate degree of
physical fitness, and (2) those who are classified as cardiac patients (anginal,
postinfarct, postoperative) who, through a period of participation in the
Monday-Wednesday-Friday program, have demonstrated a desirable degree
of cardiovascular rehabilitation and resulting physical fitness.

Exercise sessions for the Advanced Cardiac Group are conducted identically
to the Monday-Wednesday-Friday program, with the exception that a physician is not present during exercise sessions. Also, the patient receives a
physician-supervised laboratory evaluation every six months, in contrast to
the present schedule of three months. Assignment of a patient to the Advanced Cardiac Group is made only upon formal approval from the patient's
referring physician.

Your patient, _____, has recently been selected as a possible
participant in the Advanced Cardiac Group. Would you please complete the
enclosed form and return it in the addressed envelope as soon as possible.

Please feel free to contact us if you have any questions concerning this matter.
Your cooperation concerning the Cardiac Rehabilitation Program is appreciated.

Figure 65   171

Fig. 65.   Transfer Form, Physician

Patient's Name: _____Date: _____
                        Last   First   Initial

Check one of the below:

____   I consent to the transfer of my patient to the *Advanced Cardiac Group* of the Cardiac Rehabilitation Program, involving nonphysician-supervised exercise sessions twice weekly (Tuesday-Thursday).

____   I do not consent to the transfer of my patient to the *Advanced Cardiac Group* of the Cardiac Rehabilitation Program.

Signed: _____
                        (Physician)

Type or print
name of physician _____

Return to: Program Director

Fig. 66.   Transfer Letter, Patient

TO: Patient
FROM: Program Director

As you are most likely aware, in addition to the Monday-Wednesday-Friday physician-supervised aspect of the Cardiac Rehabilitation Program, there is a Tuesday-Thursday nonphysician-supervised program for those who have adequately progressed to the point of such participation. Based upon your performance in the exercise sessions and data collected during your laboratory evaluations, an invitation is now being extended to you to become a participant in the Advanced Cardiac Group.

The Advanced Cardiac Group is conducted identically to the Monday-Wednesday-Friday program in which you have been participating, with the exception that a physician is not present during exercise sessions. Also, you will receive a physician-supervised laboratory evaluation every six months, in contrast to the present schedule of three months.

Your physician is presently being contacted for his approval of your promotion to the Advanced Group, and final transfer depends upon such approval. Please complete the enclosed form and return it as soon as possible in the enclosed, addressed envelope.

Please feel free to contact the Program Director of the Cardiac Rehabilitation Program if you have any questions concerning this matter.

Figure 67   173

Fig. 67.   Transfer Form, Patient

Patient's Name _____Date _____

Please indicate your decision below:

____   I would like to participate in the Advanced Cardiac Group of the Cardiac Rehabilitation Program beginning _____.

      a. Nonphysician-supervised exercise sessions, twice weekly (Tues.-Thurs.)

      b. Physician-supervised laboratory evaluations twice yearly (every six months)

      If an accident, injury or medical complication resulting from the exercise sessions should occur, I will not consider the involved Exercise Assistant, Program Director, Board members of the Cardiac Rehabilitation Program or the involved medical institutions as being in any way responsible unless negligence on the part of that person(s) or institution is in evidence.

____   I do not wish to continue as a participant in the Cardiac Rehabilitation Program.

_____

Patient's signature   Date

_____

Program Director   Date

Return to Program Director

Fig. 68.   Re-Referral Form

Patient's Name _____Date _____

Address _____Tel. _____
           Street   City   State   Zip

Date of exercise session _____

        YOU RECOMMEND:

____ 1. Discontinue participation in the Cardiac Rehabilitation Program.
____ 2. Temporarily discontinue participation in the Cardiac Rehabilitation
          Program while further investigative procedures are being
          conducted. Probable date of reparticipation: _____.
____ 3. Continue participation in the Cardiac Rehabilitation Program
          while further investigative procedures are being conducted. Prob-
          able date of completion of investigative procedures: _____ .
____ 4. Continue participation in the Cardiac Rehabilitation Program. No
          further investigative procedures to be conducted.

Physician's Name _____Date _____

Physician's Signature _____

Incident Description:

Return to Program Director

Figure 69   175

Fig. 69A.   Monthly Exercise Session Reports
(Beginning Group—Pool)

Date _____

Name of Participant _____Example #1__ Address _____
Referring Physician _____ Clinic or Hospital _____

Weight Control	Initial Weight:	190 lbs.	(86 kg.)
	Desirable Weight:	175 lbs.	(80 kg.)
	Present Weight:	188 lbs.	(85 kg.)
	You are overweight by	13 lbs.	(6 kg.)

Exercise Prescription
Prescribed Exercise HR: 108 (18 per 10 sec.)
Actual Exercise HR: 96 (16 per 10 sec.)
Difference: in HR: 12 (2 per 10 sec.)

Exercise Tolerance (Distance)
Initial Daily Average Distance   480 yards
Present Daily Average Distance   600 yards
Initial Monthly Total Distance   6240 yards
Present Monthly Total Distance   7200 yards

Attendance
Total Exercise Sessions This Month: 13
Exercise Sessions Present: 12
Exercise Sessions Absent: 1
Attendance Percentage: 92%
Your attendance is   Satisfactory

If you have any questions, please contact me with this report.

Program Director
Cardiac Rehabilitation Program

Fig. 69B.   Monthly Exercise Session Reports
(Beginning Group—Track)

Date _____

Name of Participant _____Example #2___ Address _____
Referring Physician _____ Clinic or Hospital _____

Weight Control	Initial Weight:	160 lbs.	(73 kg.)
	Desirable Weight:	160 lbs.	(73 kg.)
	Present Weight:	160 lbs.	(73 kg.)
	You are overweight by	0 lbs.	(0 kg.)

Exercise Prescription	Prescribed Exercise HR:	120 (20 per 10 sec.)
	Actual Exercise HR:	120 (20 per 10 sec.)
	Difference: in HR:	0

Exercise Tolerance (Distance)	Initial Daily Average Distance	1.8 miles
	Present Daily Average Distance	2.1 miles
	Initial Monthly Total Distance	18.0 miles
	Present Monthly Total Distance	20.8 miles
	Grand Total Distance	34.8 miles

Attendance	Total Exercise Sessions This Month:	13
	Exercise Sessions Present:	8
	Exercise Sessions Absent:	5
	Attendance Percentage:	61%
	Your attendance is	Unsatisfactory

If you have any questions, please contact me with this report.

Program Director
Cardiac Rehabilitation Program

Figure 69   177

**Fig. 69C.   Monthly Exercise Session Reports
(Advanced Group—Track)**

Date _____

Name of Participant ____Example #3__ Address _____
Referring Physician _____ Clinic or Hospital _____

Weight Control   Initial Weight: 240 lbs.   (109 kg.)
                                    Desirable Weight: 185 lbs.   (84 kg.)
                                    Present Weight: 190 lbs.   (86 kg.)
                                    You are overweight by   5 lbs.   (2 kg.)

Exercise Prescription   Prescribed Exercise HR: 144 (24 per 10 sec.)
                                    Actual Exercise HR: 138 (23 per 10 sec.)
                                    Difference in HR: 6 (1 per 10 sec.)

Exercise Tolerance (Distance)   Initial Daily Average Distance   1.7 miles
                                    Present Daily Average Distance   3.0 miles
                                    Initial Monthly Total Distance   20.4 miles
                                    Present Monthly Total Distance   27.0 miles
                                    Grand Total Distance   243.2 miles

Attendance   Total Exercise Sessions This Month: 9
                                    Exercise Sessions Present: 9
                                    Exercise Sessions Absent: 0
                                    Attendance Percentage: 100%
                                    Your attendance is   Good

If you have any questions, please contact me with this report.

Program Director
Cardiac Rehabilitation Program

Fig. 70.   Patient's First Month Report Memo

TO: Patient
FROM: Program Director

Enclosed you will find a Monthly Progress Report relative to your first month of participation within the Cardiac Rehabilitation Program. The report provides you with information relative to (1) weight fluctuation, (2) exercise tolerance (distance traveled), (3) prescribed exercise heart rate, and (4) attendance. Each month you will receive a report with information relative to the most recent month of participation compared to your first month. Your physician also receives a copy of this report monthly.

If you have questions concerning the enclosed report, please feel free to ask for assistance from any of the program staff.

Figure 71   179

Fig. 71.   Physician's First Month Report Memo

TO: Primary Physician
FROM: Program Director
RE: Exercise Progress Report Flow Sheet

Enclosed is a copy of the revised Exercise Progress Report Flow Sheet
for _____.

You will receive a revised Exercise Report Flow Sheet each month your
patient participates in the Cardiac Rehabilitation Program.

Please feel free to contact me at your convenience if you have any
questions concerning the enclosed flow sheet, or any other aspect of the
Cardiac Rehabilitation Program.

Date: _____

Fig. 72.   Subsequent Monthly Reports, Participant and Physician Memo

TO: Patients and Referring Physicians, Cardiac Rehabilitation Program
FROM: Program Director

    Enclosed you will find the Exercise Session Progress Report(s) for the last month. The report provides information relative to: (1) weight fluctuation, (2) exercise tolerance (distance traveled), (3) prescribed exercise heart rate, and (4) attendance.
    Please feel free to contact me if you have any questions concerning this material.

Figure 73   181

Fig. 73.   Emergency CPR Procedures for Employees

A. SAFETY HINTS

1. Watch the person you are assigned to; he is your responsibility.
2. Spread out along the pool or track so that the entire area is under observation.
3. Know what your responsibilities are and review them periodically.
4. In case of emergency, don't panic—be cool and collected.

B. PRE-EXERCISE OR LABORATORY EVALUATION PROCEDURES

1. Hook up defibrillator.
2. Open up drug cabinet.
3. Have keys in immediate area.
4. Know your "Assignment of Responsibility."

C. RESPONSIBILITIES

1. **Call Physician**—2 people.
   Contact physician if he is not in your immediate area.
2. **Call ambulance**—1 person.
   Know the location of phones immediately accessible from the pool area, track area, and laboratory evaluation area. If access to phones requires keys to specific offices, know where or from whom to obtain these keys.

   Call should be placed to the following number: _____.

   The following information should be given: "This is an emergency. I am calling from the Cardiac Rehabilitation Program at _____. We have a cardiac stretcher case to be rushed to the hospital. Report to (closest location to patient)."

   Talk slowly and distinctly. Upon completing call, proceed to arrival location of ambulance and direct attendants to patient.
3. **Rescue Team**—3 people.
   Get the patient out of the water or off the track and onto a stretcher.

The American Heart Association has established the following steps to be taken in the event of an apparent cardiac arrest:

1. Establish unresponsiveness (4 to 10 seconds). Shake patient's shoulders, shout "Are you OK?"
2. Tilt patient's head, open airway (1 to 2 seconds).
3. Take patient's pulse (5 to 10 seconds). (Maintain tilted head position with one hand and feel carotid pulse with other hand.)
4. Precordial thump—midsternum.

5. Give four ventilations (3 to 5 seconds).
6. Palpate pulse again (as in step 3 above).
7. If no pulse, start compressions and ventilations (five compressions followed by one ventilation with two rescuers).
   Rescuer No. 1 Strike a blow to the sternum and begin heart massage. Depress the chest five times to each forceful entrance of air into the patient's lungs.
   Rescuer No. 2 Give mouth-to-mouth resuscitation.
   Rescuer No. 3 Raise the legs of the patient as previously instructed.
4. **Stretcher**—1 person.
   Get the stretcher and bring it to the area where the patient is located.
5. **Drying Off**—1 person.
   This person will be responsible for drying off the patient after he has been removed from the water. (Swimming pool only.)
6. **Defibrillator**—1 person.
   This person will be responsible for moving the defibrillator to the area where the patient is located. (Know location of all outlets in the area.)
7. **Exercise-Take Charge**—1 person.
   Responsible for continuing exercise program with other patients away from the emergency area.

D.   GENERAL INFORMATION

1. Do not initiate the foregoing procedures unless the patient is actually in need of emergency care. The closest individual and/or the Attending Physician will make this decision and will indicate that an emergency situation exists by swinging an arm above his or her head. There will be situations when a participant will feel weak, faint, or have chest pain. Contact the physician when such a situation arises.
2. The remaining participants are to continue to exercise. This is the responsibility of the Laboratory-Exercise Assistants who are not involved in the emergency procedures.

Figure 74   183

Fig. 74.   General CPR Protocol

I. Make assignments before exercise session begins. Make sure each person understands his responsibilities. It is a good idea to frequently test and question staff on their responsibilities.

II. The assignments include:
    A. Basic life support, given by CPR-certified individual
    B. Initiate advance life support—CPR
        1. Get physician.
        2. Get defibrillator.
        3. Call ambulance.
        4. Get drugs and oxygen ready for use.
        5. Get patients together and continue to exercise somewhere away from the emergency.

Fig. 75.   CPR in Swimming Pool Area

1. Exercise Leader (Pool) will make sure that CPR sheets have been signed by staff for CPR assignments.
2. Have staff sign in and make sure each individual knows and understands his responsibilities in case of an emergency.
3. If defibrillation is necessary, patient will be taken into the hallway and placed on the wooden rack.
4. Hold practice sessions at least once a week.

Figure 76   185

Fig. 76.   CPR in Track Area

1. Exercise Leader (Track, Exercise) will make sure that CPR sheets have been signed by staff for CPR assignments.
2. Have staff sign in and make sure each individual knows and understands his responsibilities.
3. Hold practice sessions at least once a week.

Fig. 77.   CPR in Locker Room

1. Two (2) staff members (with AHA-approved CPR certification) will report to the locker room at the end of the exercise session (6:00) and stay there until the last individual leaves the locker room.
2. Two (2) males in the men's locker rooms and two (2) females in the women's locker rooms will be designated by a monthly CPR locker room roster. These are the individuals who are assigned CPR duty in the locker rooms.
3. Encourage patients to take warm showers and not hot or cold showers.
4. In case of an emergency, one individual will perform CPR while the other individual will get help and direct people to the proper CPR procedures (check CPR protocol).

Figure 78 187

Fig. 78. CPR Sign in Sheet

DATE: _____ 19_____. DAY OF THE WEEK: _____

Exercise Leaders, please sign below.

Return this sheet to Human Performance Laboratory after exercise session. (Initials only.)

Student Help:	Time:	Student Help:	Time:	Volunteers:	Time:
_____	_____	_____		_____	
_____	_____	_____		_____	
_____	_____	_____		_____	
_____	_____	_____		_____	
_____	_____	_____		_____	
_____	_____	_____		_____	
_____	_____	_____		_____	
_____	_____	_____		_____	
_____	_____	_____		_____	
_____	_____	_____		_____	
_____	_____	_____		_____	
_____	_____	_____		_____	

CPR Duty:
1. Perform CPR _____ (CPR Certified)
2. Summon Doctor
3. Get Defibrillator
4. Get Drug Box
5. CALL Ambulance

Fig. 79.   Portable LifePak/33 Defibrillator.   Check-Out Procedures

A. The following procedures will be done on a daily basis (Monday through
   Friday), once at 4:45 p.m. and once at 6:00 p.m.
   1. Unplug charger from unit.
   2. Turn main power control ON. Green light should come on.
   3. Make sure defibrillator "Watt-Seconds" control is OFF.
   4. Touch one paddle. Interference should appear on scope. Repeat with
      the other paddle.
   5. Place paddles together. Interference should disappear on scope.
   6. Turn defibrillator "Watt-Seconds" control ON and set at approxi-
      mately 25 watt-seconds. Place paddles firmly together and depress
      both buttons. Defibrillator meter should drop to zero instantly and a
      "thump" should be heard. PADDLES SHOULD NOT BE DIS-
      CHARGED TOGETHER ABOVE 50 WATT-SECONDS.

   7. *4:45 p.m. Protocol*
      Obtain the defibrillator test cone from the Human Performance Lab.
      Turn defibrillator to 200 watt-seconds, press "recharge" button.
      Green light should stay on and meter should reach 200 watt-seconds
      within ten seconds. Make sure test cone is on a wooden-based table.
      Place paddles on each side of the defibrillator test cone on the round
      metal plates. Paddles must touch the metal plates firmly. Do *not* fire
      defibrillator in the air.
      Push buttons simultaneously. Defibrillator should discharge. You
      should hear a thump, and the indicator for watt-seconds will drop back
      to zero.

   6:00 p.m. Protocol
      Obtain the defibrillator test cone from the Human Performance Lab.
      Turn defibrillator to 200 watt-seconds, press "recharge" button. Green
      light should stay on and meter should reach 200 watt-seconds within
      ten seconds. Press "To 400 Watt-Seconds" until meter indicates 400
      watt-seconds. Make sure test cone is on a wooden based table. Place
      paddles on each side of the defibrillator test cone on the round metal
      plates. Paddles must touch the metal plates firmly. Do *not* fire defibril-
      lator in the air.
      Push buttons simultaneously. Defibrillator should discharge. You
      should hear a thump, and the indicator for watt-seconds will drop back
      to zero.
   8. Shut off "Watt-Seconds" control. Shut off main power switch.
   9. Replace paddles on handle of unit.
   10. Plug charger back into unit. Red light should come on.

Figure 79   189

B. Who will perform task:
    Monday-Wednesday-Friday—Exercise Leader in charge of track.
    Tuesday-Thursday—Exercise Leader in charge of Tuesday-Thursday
    programs.
    Responsible individual will not have someone else perform the task. The
    defibrillator can be extremely dangerous when not used properly.

C. If defibrillator is functioning properly, individual will initial defibrillator
    daily test sheet on the respective date. Necessary information required by
    the test sheet will also be submitted. If the defibrillator is not functioning
    properly, notify the Program Director.

Fig. 80.   Portable LifePak/33 Defibrillator Daily Test Sheet

Month of _____ 19 ___

Date	4:45 p.m.			6:00 p m.		
	Initials	Delivered Wattage	Charge OK (Yes or No)	Initials	Delivered Wattage	Charge OK (Yes or No)
1						
2						
3						
4						
5						
6						
7						
8						
9						
10						
11						
12						
13						
14						
15						
16						
17						
18						
19						
20						
21						
22						
23						
24						
25						
26						
27						
28						
29						
30						
31						

Figure 81   191

Fig. 81.   Nonportable Defibrillator (Large "Plug-in") Check-Out Procedures

1. The following procedures will be utilized at 2:00 p.m. on the day of the Laboratory Evaluation:
   a. Obtain defibrillator test cone from the Human Performance Laboratory.
   b. Turn defibrillator power "on." Light will come on.
   c. Put paddles together.
   d. Establish desired watts per second by pressing maroon button in the middle of the console.
   e. Place paddles on each side of the defibrillator test cone on the round metal plates. Make sure cone is on a wooden based table. Paddles must touch the metal plates firmly. Do *not* fire the defibrillator in the air.
   f. Push both buttons on the paddles simultaneously. Defibrillator should discharge. Test light on left top corner should blink, and you should hear a thump. The delivered watt-seconds indicator will immediately go down to approximately zero.
   g. Turn power off.
   h. Replace paddles on top of defibrillator. Make sure you place the paddles facing up in the air; otherwise, you will scratch the surface of the paddles.
2. Who will perform task: Head Laboratory Technician No. 1 for that particular month.
   Responsible individual will *not* have someone else perform the task. The defibrillator is extremely dangerous when not used properly.
3. If defibrillator is functioning properly, individual will initial defibrillator daily test sheet on the respective date. Necessary information required by the sheet will also be submitted. If the defibrillator is not functioning properly, notify the Program Director.

Fig. 82.   Nonportable Defibrillator Daily Test Sheet

Month of _____ 19 ___

Date	Initials	Delivered Wattage	Charge OK (Yes or No)
1			
2			
3			
4			
5			
6			
7			
8			
9			
10			
11			
12			
13			
14			
15			
16			
17			
18			
19			
20			
21			
22			
23			
24			
25			
26			
27			
28			
29			
30			
31			

Figure 83   193

Fig. 83

General Education Program of the La Crosse Cardiac Rehabilitation Program

"Nutrition and Holiday Entertaining"

Thursday, December 16, 1976
7:30 - 9:00 pm
Indian Commons, Cartwright Center

University of Wisconsin - La Crosse Campus
Open to the public - no admission charge.

Sue Murvich, M·S·, Clinical Nutritionist, Gunderson Clinic and
Consulting Nutritionist, La Crosse Cardiac Rehabilitation Program

Refreshments will be served

How to prepare holiday meals without increasing the risk factors for coronary heart disease.

Fig. 84

General Education Program of the La Crosse
Cardiac Rehabilitation Program

STRESS
REDUCTION
CLINIC

With Dr. Jack Curtis, Ph. D., Assistant Professor, Department of Health
Education, University of Wisconsin-LaCrosse

WHY: Stress is often considered a risk factor to Coronary Heart Disease

WHO: Open to the public

WHEN: January 27, 29, Feb 3, 10, 19 & 24.
            Participants must attend all seven sessions

TIME: 7:00 - 8:15 p.m.

Where: Room 26, Mitchell Hall, University of Wisconsin-LaCrosse

Cost: $20.00 with $10.00 refunded upon successful completion of the program

            Enrollment is limited, with participants in the LaCrosse Cardiac
            Rehabilitation program receiving first priority in registering.
            Another clinic will be held in March. People who are turned
            away from the first clinic will be given priority in signing
            up for the second clinic.

How: Send application and check to:
            LaCrosse Cardiac Rehab Program
            132 Mitchell Hall
            University of Wisc-LaCrosse
            LaCrosse, Wisconsin 54601

            Make checks payable to:
            Univ. of Wisc-LaCrosse, Cardiac Rehab

I am interested in participating in the stress reduction clinic to be held on Jan. 27, 29, Feb. 3, 10, 19 & 24. Enclosed is a check for $20.00
Name_____
Address_____
_____
Telephone #_____
I am presently participating in the LaCrosse Cardiac Rehab Program. Please check
_____yes   No

Figure 85   195

Fig. 85

General Education Program of the La Crosse
Cardiac Rehabilitation Program

Smoke Termination

Clinic

With Dr. Gary Gilmore, Ph. D., Assistant Professor, Community Health, UWEX, and Department of Health Education, University of Wisconsin-LaCrosse.

WHY: Death rates from heart attacks in men range from 50 to 200% higher among cigarette smokers than among non-smokers. Smoking is considered a risk factor to Coronary Heart Disease.

WHO: Anyone who smokes and wants to stop. Open to the public.

When: January 7, 14, 21 & 28, 1976.
Participants must attend all four sessions.

Time: 7:00 - 8:30 p.m.

Where: Room 26, Mitchell Hall, University of Wisconsin-LaCrosse

Cost: $5.00 with the full amount refunded upon successful completion of the program.

Enrollment is limited with participants in the LaCrosse Cardiac Rehabilitation program receiving first priority in registering. Another clinic will be held later in the year. People who are turned away from this first clinic will be given priority in the second clinic.

How: Send application and check to:
LaCrosse Cardiac Rehab Program
132 Mitchell Hall
University of Wisc-LaCrosse
LaCrosse, Wisc 54601

Make checks payable to:
Univ of Wisc-Lacrosse, Cardiac Rehab

I am interested in participating in the smoke termination clinic to be held on Jan. 7, 14, 21 & 28. Enclosed is a check for $5.00.

Name_____

Address_____

_____

Telephone # _____

I am presently participating in the LaCrosse Cardiac Rehab Program. please check
_____ yes   _____ No

Fig. 86

Patient Education Program of the La Crosse

Cardiac Rehabilitation Program

CROSS-COUNTRY

SKI CLINIC

With Ms. Betsy Clark, M.S., Instructor, Department of Physical Education, University of Wisconsin-La Crosse and Cross Country Ski Instructor at Tommy's River Forest Ski Area, Galesville, Wisconsin.

WHO: ADVANCED (T - TH) Cardiac Rehabilitation Program Participants and Family
Adult Physical Fitness Program Participants and Family

WHY: You should consider some other alternatives to supplement your running. Cross-country skiing is presently one of the fastest growing winter sports in this country. It is fun and inexpensive when compared to downhill skiing. Cross-country skiing is for all ages, a fantastic family affair activity.

WHEN: Monday, January 24; Wednesday, January 26; Monday, January 31; Wednesday, February 2. Participants must attend all four (4) sessions.

WHERE: Meet in Room 119, Mitchell Hall

TIME: 4:30 - 6:00 p.m.

COST: Free - if you have equipment.
Arrangements have been made with Motorless Motion, 1914 Campbell Road (across the street from the Human Performance Lab) to rent cross-country skis. Total cost will be $6.00. If interested in renting submit the equipment rental form to the Rehab. office by 4:30 p.m. January 20, 1977. There are only a limited amount of cross-country ski rentals. If renting, you are responsible for obtaining the equipment, payment and returning them each day immediately after the Clinic.

HOW: If you are interested in participating, you must pre-register by filling in the enclosed form and returning it to the Rehab. office by January 20, 1977, by 4:30 p.m.

Appendix

appendix A
Bibliography

ADMINISTRATION

Policies and Procedures of the LaCrosse Cardiac Rehabilitation Program, University of Wisconsin-LaCrosse, 1974.

Cooper, J., and Willig, S.: Nonphysicians for coronary care delivery: are they legal? Am. J. Cardiol., *28(3)*:363–365, September, 1971.

Herbert, W., and Herbert, D.: Exercise testing in adults: legal procedural considerations for the physical educator and exercise specialist. JOHPER, *46(6)*:17–18, June, 1975.

Kasch, F., and Boyer, J.: *Adult Fitness: Principles and Practices*. Greely, Colorado: All American Productions and Publications, 1968.

McNiece, H.F.: Legal aspects of exercise testing. N.Y. State J. Med., *72*:1822–1824, July 15, 1972.

McNiece, H.F.: The legal basis for awards in cardiac cases. N. Y. State J. Med., *61*:906–912, March 15, 1961.

Van der Smissen: Legal aspects of adult fitness programs. JOHPER, *45(2)*:55–56, 1974.

Wilmore, J.: Organization and administration guidelines for adult fitness programs. JOHPER, *45(2)*:45, 1974.

Wilson, P.: Cardiac Rehabilitation Programs. JOHPER, *45(2)*:47, 1974.

BEHAVIORAL, PSYCHOLOGIC, AND SOCIAL MODIFICATIONS

Adsett, C.A., and Bruhn, J.G.: Short-term group psychotherapy in post-MI patients and their wives. Can. Med. Assoc. J., *99*:577, 1968.

198

Appendix   199

Arthur, R.J.: Masters swimming program stimulates fitness motivation. Phys. and
     Sports Med., *4(10)*:63–66, 1976.
Bilodeau, C.B., and Hackett, T.P.: Issues raised in a group setting by patients
     recovering from myocardial infarction. Am. J. Psychiat., *128*:73, 1971.
Bruhn, J.G., Wolf, S., and Philips, B.V.: Depression and death in myocardial
     infarction: a psychosocial study of screening male coronary patients over nine
     years. J. Psychosom. Res., *15*:305, 1971.
Cassem, N.H., and Hackett, T.P.: Psychiatric consultation in a coronary care unit.
     Ann. Intern. Med., *75*:9, 1971.
Cay, E.L., et al.: Psychological reactions to a coronary care unit. J. Psych. Res.,
     16:425, 1972.
Croog, S.H., and LeVine, S.: After the heart attack: social aspects of rehabilitation.
     Medical Insight, *5(9)*, October, 1973.
Croog, S.H., Shapiro, D.S., and LeVine, S.: Denial among male heart patients.
     Psychosom. Med., *33(5)*:385–397, 1971.
Davis, M.S.: Physiologic, psychological and demographic factors in patient
     compliance with doctors' orders. Med. Care, *6*:115, 1968.
Dixon, R.G., Jr.: *Social Security Disability and Mass Justice. A Problem in Welfare
     Adjudication.* New York: Praeger Publications, 1973.
Foster, S., and Andreoli, K.: The postcoronary patient. Behavior following acute
     myocardial infarction. Am. J. Nurs., *70*:2344, 1970.
Friedman, M., and Rosenman, R.: *Type A Behavior and Your Heart.* Greenwich,
     Conn.: Fawcett Publications Inc., 1975.
Groden, B.M., and Brown, R.F.: Differential psychological effects of early and late
     mobilization after myocardial infarction. Scand. J. Rehabil. Med., *2*:60–64,
     1970.
Guild, W.R.: *After Your Heart Attack.* New York; Harper & Row Publishers, 1969.
Hackett, T.P., et al.: Blue collar and white collar responses to having heart attack.
     Psychology Society, National Meeting, Boston: 1972.
Hackett, T.P., Cassem, N.H., and Wishnie, H.A.: The coronary care unit: an
     appraisal of its psychological hazards. New Eng. J. Med., *279*:1365, 1968.
Hackett, T.P., and Weisman, A.D.: Denial as factor in patients with heart disease
     and cancer. Ann. N. Y. Acad. Sci., *164*:802, 1969.
Henry, J.P., and Cassel, J.C.: Psychosocial factors in essential hypertension; recent
     epidemiologic and animal experimental evidence. Am. J. Epidemiol., *90*:171–
     200, 1971.
Holmes, T.H., and Rahe, R.H.: The social readjustment rating scale. J. Psychosom.
     Res., *11*:213–218, 1967.
Howell, M.L., and Alderman, R.B.: Psychological determinants of fitness. Can.
     Med. Assoc. J., *96*:721–728, 1967.
Jenkins, C.D.: Psychologic and social precursors of coronary disease. New Eng. J.
     Med., *284*:244, 307, 1971.
Kong-Ming New, P., et al.: The support structure of heart and stroke patients: a
     study of significant others in patient rehabilitation. Soc. Sci. Med., *2*:185, 1968.
Lawton, G.: *Straight to the Heart.* New York: International Universities Press Inc.,
     1956.
Mechanic, D.: Social and psychological factors affecting the presentation of bodily
     complaints. N. Engl. J. Med., *286*:1132, 1972.

Mordkoff, A.M., and Parsons, O.A.: The coronary personality—a critique. Int. J. Psychiat., *5*:413, 1968.

Powers, M.: Emotional aspects of cardiovascular surgery. Cardiovasc. Nursing, *4(2)*:7–10, March-April, 1968.

Rahe, R.H., et al.: Group therapy in the outpatient management of post-myocardial infarction patients. Psychiatry Med., *4*:77, 1973.

Rotter, J.B.: Generalized expectancies for internal versus external control of reinforcement. Psych. Monographs, *80 (No. 1, Whole No. 609)*:1–28, 1966.

Safilios-Rothschild, C.: *The Sociology and Social Psychology of Disability and Rehabilitation.* New York: Random House, 1970.

Strauss, R.: Social change and the rehabilitation concept. In *Sociology and Rehabilitation,* ed. by M.B. Sussman. Washington, D.C.: American Sociological Association, 1966.

Taggart, P., Parkinson, P., and Carruthers, M.: Cardiac responses to thermal, physical and emotional stress. Br. Med. J., *3*:71–76, July 8, 1972.

Wardwell, W.I., and Bahnson, C.B.: Behavioral variables and myocardial infarction in the southeastern Connecticut heart study. J. Chronic. Dis., *26*:447, 1973.

Weis, E., et al.: Emotional factors in coronary occlusion. Arch. Intern. Med., *99*:628–640, 1957.

Wolf, S.: Emotional stress and the heart. J. Rehabil., *32*:42–45, 1966.

Young, R.J., and Ismail, A.H.: Personality differences of adult men before and after a physical fitness program. Res. Qtr., *47(3)*:513–519, 1976.

Zohman, B.L.: Managing emotional problems called major consideration in treating post-M.I. patient. Clin. Trends Cardiol., *1(4)*:1–7, 1972.

Zung, W.W.: Evaluating treatment methods for depressive disorders. Am. J. Psychiatry, *124*:40–48, 1968.

Zung, W.W., Richards, C.G., Gables, C., and Short, M.: Self-rating depression scale in an outpatient clinic. Arch. Gen. Psychiatry, *13*:508–515, 1965.

DIABETES, HEART DISEASE AND EXERCISE

Harris, P., et al.: The metabolism of glucose during exercise in patients with rheumatic heart disease. Clin. Sci., *23:*561–569, 1962.

Klachko, D.M., et al.: Blood glucose levels during walking in normal and diabetic subjects. Diabetes, *21(2)*:89–100, 1972.

Levitas, I.M., and Kristac, J.J.: Stress exercise testing of the young diabetic for the detection of unknown coronary artery disease. Juvenile Diabetes, *8(6)*:845, June, 1972.

Vikhert, A.M., Zhdanov, V.S., and Matova, E.E.: Atherosclerosis of the aorta and coronary arteries in patients with ischemic heart disease associated with hypertension and diabetes mellitus. Kardiologiya, *12*:40–46, 1972. (Eng. Summ.)

ELECTROCARDIOGRAPHY

Anderson, G.J., and Blieden, M.F.: The high frequency electrocardiogram in coronary artery disease. Am. Heart J., *89*:340–358, 1975.

Barnard, J., et al.: Cardiovascular responses to sudden strenuous exercise—heart rate, blood pressure, and EKG. J. Appl. Physiol., *34(6)*:833–837, 1973.

Beckwith, J.: *Clinical Electrocardiography.* New York: McGraw-Hill, 1970.

Blackburn, H., and Katigbak, R.: What electrocardiographic leads to take after exercise? Am. Heart J., *67*:184, 1964.

Blackburn, H.: The exercise electrocardiogram: differences in interpretation. Am. J. Cardiol., *21*:871–880, 1968.

Blackburn, H.: Importance of the electrocardiogram in populations outside the hospital. Can. Med. Assoc. J., *108*:1262–1265, 1973.

Blackburn, H., et al.: *Measurement in Exercise Electrocardiography.* Springfield, Ill.: Charles C Thomas, 1959.

Blomqvist, G.: The Frank lead exercise electrocardiogram: a quantitative study based on averaging technique and digital computer analysis. Acta Med. Scand. Suppl., *440*:5–98, 1965.

Bruce, R.A.: Exercise electrocardiography. In *The Heart,* ed. by J.W. Hurst. 3rd ed. New York: McGraw-Hill, 1974.

Burch, G.E.: *A Primer of Cardiology.* Philadelphia: Lea & Febiger, 1971.

Burch, G.E.: *A Primer of Electrocardiography.* Philadelphia: Lea & Febiger, 1972.

Butler, H.H.: *How to Read an ECG.* Albany: Delmar Publishers, 1975.

Chahine, R.A., Raizner, A.E., and Ishimori, T.: The clinical significance of exercise-induced ST-segment elevation. Circulation, *54(2)*:209–212, 1976.

Cohn, P.F., Vokonas, P.S., Herman, M.V., and Gorlin, R.: Postexercise electrocardiogram in patients with abnormal resting electrocardiograms. Circulation, *43*:648, 1971.

Dimond, E.G.: *The Exercise Electrocardiogram in Office Practice.* Springfield, Ill.: Charles C Thomas, 1961.

Dower, G.E.: A lead synthesizer for the Frank system to simulate the standard 12-lead electrocardiogram. Electrocardiology, *1*:101–116, 1968.

Dubin, D.: *Rapid Interpretation of EKGs.* Tampa: Cover Publishers, 1974.

Eddleman, E.E.: Examination of precordial movements. In *The Heart.* ed. by J.W. Hurst. 3rd ed. New York: McGraw-Hill, 1974.

The Electrocardiogram in Hypertension. Merck Sharp & Dohme, Division of Merck & Company, Inc., West Point, Pa. 19486.

Friesinger, G., et al.: Exercise ECG and vasoregulatory abnormalities. Am. J. Cardiol., *30*:733–738, 1972.

Hashimoto, K., et al.: Significance of ST-segment elevations in acute myocardial ischemia. Am. J. Cardiol., *37*:493–500, 1976.

Jacobs, W., Brattle, W., and Ronari, J.: False positive ST-T wave changes secondary to hyperventilation and exercise: a cineangiographic correlation. Ann. Intern. Med., *81(4)*:479–482, 1974.

Kannel, W.B., Gordon, T., Offutt, D.: Left ventricular hypertrophy by electrocardiogram, prevalence, incidence and mortality in the Framingham study. Ann. Intern. Med., *71*:89–105, 1969.

Karatun, O.: Axis deviation of the heart on fit and unfit subjects and possible effect of interval training. Unpublished Master's Thesis, Univ. of Kansas, 1972, p. 42–58.

Kattus, A.A., Jorgensen, C.R., Worden, R.E., and Alvaro, A.B.: ST-segment depression with near maximal exercise in detection of pre-clinical coronary heart disease. Circulation, *54*:585–594, 1971.

Lary, B., and Goldschlager: Electrocardiographic changes during hyperventilation: resembling myocardial ischemia in patients with normal arteriograms. Am. Heart J., *87(3)*:383–390, 1974.

Likoff, W., et al.: Coronary arteriography: correlation with electrocardiographic response to measured exercise. Am. J. Cardiol., *18*:160, 1966.

Likoff, W.: Echocardiography: It's here to stay. Clin. Trends Cardiol., Sept.-Oct., 1976.

Lynn, T.N., and Wolf, S.: The prognostic significance of the ballistocardiogram in ischemic heart disease. Am. Heart J., *88*:277–280. 1974.

Mason, R.E., Likar, I., Biern, R.O., and Ross, R.S.: Multiple lead exercise electrocardiography. Experience in 107 normal subjects and 67 patients with angina pectoris, and comparison with coronary cine-arteriography in 84 patients. Circulation, *34*:517–522, 1967.

McCohonay, D.R., McCalister, B.O., and Smith, R.E.: Post exercise electrocardiography: correlation with coronary arteriography and L.V. hemodynamics. Am. J. Cardiol., *28*:1–9, 1971.

Miller, R.R., Massumi, R.A., and Mason, D.T.: The resting electrocardiogram in assessing ischemic heart disease. Geriatrics, *30*:51–57, 1975.

Most, A.S., Kemp, H.G., and Gorlin, R.: Postexercise electrocardiography in patients with arteriographically documented coronary artery disease. Ann. Intern. Med., *71*:1043, 1969.

Murayama, M., et al.: Studies on the lead system for telemetering the exercise electrocardiogram. Jap. Heart J., *5*:312, 1964.

Pardee, H.E.B.: An electrocardiographic sign of coronary occlusion. Arch. Int. Med., *26*:244, 1920.

Phillips, R., and Feeney, M.: *The Cardiac Rhythms, A Systematic Approach to Interpretation.* Philadelphia: W. B. Saunders Company, 1973.

Rautaharju, P.M., et al.: Computer analysis of the exercise electrocardiogram. In *Electrical Activity of the Heart.* ed. by G.W. Manning and S.P. Ahuja. Springfield, Ill.: Charles C Thomas, 1969.

Rautaharju, P.M., and Blackburn, H.: The exercise electrocardiogram: experience in analysis of "noisy" cardiograms with a small computer. Am. Heart J., *69*:515, 1965.

Robb, G.P., and Marks, H.H.: Post exercise electrocardiogram in arteriosclerotic heart disease. JAMA, *200*:918–926, 1967.

Rosner, S.W., et al.: A computer analysis of the exercise electrocardiogram. Am. J. Cardiol., *20*:356, 1967.

Schiffer, F., et al.: The quiz electrocardiogram: a new diagnostic and research technique for evaluating the relation between emotional stress and ischemic heart disease. Am. J. Cardiol., *37*:41–47, 1976.

Schrueden, R., and Suedhoff, H.: *Practical Evaluation of the Electrocardiogram.* Springfield, Ill.: Charles C Thomas, 1969.

Sheffield, L.T., et al.: On-line analysis of the exercise electrocardiogram. Circulation, *40*:935, 1969.

Simonson, E., and Keys, A.: The effect of an ordinary meal on the electrocardiogram. Circulation, *1*:1000–5, 1950.

Simoons, M.L., and Hugenholtz, P.G.: Gradual changes of ECG waveform during and after exercise in normal subjects. Circulation, *52*:570–576, 1975.

Smith, R.F., and Wherry, R.J., Jr.: Quantitative interpretation of the exercise electrocardiogram. Circulation, *34*:1044, 1966.
Stuart, R.J.: Upsloping ST-segments in exercise stress testing. Am. J. Cardiol., *37*:19–22, 1976.

EMERGENCY PROCEDURES

Standards for cardiopulmonary resuscitation (CPR) and emergency cardiac care. Supplement to JAMA, *227(7)*:18, 1974.
Program yourself to start a heart; meet the professor! Emergency Medicine, *3 (11)*:106–124, November, 1971.
Goldberger, E.: *Treatment of Cardiac Emergencies*. St. Louis: C.V. Mosby Company, 1974.
Grace, W.J., Kennedy, R., and Nolte, C.: Blind defibrillation. Am. J. Cardiol., *34(1)*:115–116, 1974.
Hackett, T.P., and Cassem, N.H.: Factors contributing to delay in responding to the signs and symptoms of acute myocardial infarction. Am. J. Cardiol., *24*:651, 1969.
Pyfer, H., and Doane, B.: Cardiac arrest during exercise training: report of successfully treated CAS attributed to preparedness. JAMA, *210(1)*:101–102, 1969.

ENVIRONMENTAL FACTORS

Aronow, W., Stemmer, E., and Isbell, M.: Effects of carbon monoxide exposure on intermittent claudication. Circulation, *49(3)*:415–417, 1974.
Aronow, W., et al.: Effects of cigarette smoking and breathing carbon monoxide on cardiovascular hemodynamics in anginal pain. Circulation, *50(8)*:340–347, 1974.
Astrup, P.: Carbon monoxide, smoking and cardiovascular disease. Circulation, *48(6)*:1167–1168, 1973.
Claremont, A.: Comparison of metabolic temperature, heart rate and ventilatory response to exercise at extreme ambient temperature 0–35° C. Med. Sci. Sports, *7(2)*:150–154, Summer, 1974.
Dill, D., et al.: Responses of men and women to two-hour walks in desert heat. J. Appl. Physiol., *35(2)*:231–235, 1973.
Dinman, B.: Work in hot environments: Field studies of workload, thermal stress and physiological response. J. Occup. Med., *16(12)*:785–791, 1974.
Epstein, S., et al.: Effects of a reduction in environmental temperature on circulatory response to exercise in man. N. Engl. J. Med., *2*:280–287, January, 1969.
Masher, J.T.: Effects of high-altitude exposure on submaximal endurance capacity of men. J. Appl. Physiol., *37(6)*:895–898, December, 1974.
Mostardi, R.: Effects of increased body temperature due to exercise on heart rate and maximum aerobic power. Eur. J. Appl. Physiol., *33(3)*:237–245, 1974.
Nader, E.R.: Mechanisms of thermal acclimation to exercise and heat. J. Appl. Physiol., *37(4)*:515–520. October, 1974.

Toohey, J.V.: What health educators need to know about the ecology of physical activity in a polluted environment. J. Am. Coll. Health Assoc., *23(2)*:143–145, December, 1974.

EXERCISE PHYSIOLOGY

Allen, T.E., Byrd, R.J., and Smith, D.P.: Hemodynamic consequences of circuit weight training. Res. Qtr., *47*:299–306, 1976.

Amsterdam, E.A., et al.: Response of the rat heart to strenuous exercise: physical, biochemical and functional correlates. (Abstract) Clin. Res., *20*:361, 1972.

Arcos, J.C., et al.: Changes in ultrastructure and respiratory control in mitochondria of rat heart hypertrophied by exercise. Exp. Mol. Pathol., *8*:49, 1968.

Astrand, P.O., and Rhyming, I.: Nomogram for calculation of aerobic capacity (physical fitness) from pulsenotes during sub-maximal work. J. Appl. Physiol., *7*:218, 1954.

Astrand, P., and Rodahl, K.: *Textbook of Work Physiology.* New York: McGraw-Hill Book Company, 1970.

Bevegard, S., Holmgren, A., and Johsson, B.: The effect of body position on the circulation at rest and during exercise, with special reference to the influence on the stroke volume. Acta Physiol. Scand., *49*:279–298, 1960.

Bhan, A.K., and Scheuer, J.: Effects of physical training on cardiac actomyosin adenosine triphosphate activity. Am. J. Physiol., *223*:1486–1490, 1972.

Bhan, A.K., and Scheuer, J.: Effects of physical conditioning on cardiac myosin. (Abstr) Circulation, *46(Suppl II)*:11–131, 1972.

Bing, R.J.: Coronary circulation and cardiac metabolism. In *Circulation of the Blood; Men and Ideas.* ed. by Fishman, A.P., and Richard, D.W., New York: Oxford University Press, 1964, pp. 199–264.

Bjuro, T., Sanne, H., Stenberg, J., and Varnauskas, E.: Mobilization after acute coronary infarction. In *Coronary Heart Disease and Physical Fitness.* ed. by Larsen, O.A., and Malmborg, R.O. Baltimore: University Park Press, 1971, pp. 180–182.

Blackburn, H.: Progress in the epidemiology and prevention of coronary heart disease. In *Progress in Cardiology.* 3rd ed. by Yu, P.N., and Goodwin, J.F. Philadelphia: Lea & Febiger, 1974. pp. 1–36.

Bloor, C.M., and Leon, A.S.: Interaction of age and exercise on the heart and its blood supply. Lab. Invest., *22*:160, 1970.

Bloor, C.M., Pasyk, S., and Leon, A.S.: Interaction of age and exercise on organ and cellular development. Am. J. Pathol., *58*:185, 1970.

Blomqvist, G.: Exercise physiology related to diagnosis of coronary artery disease, myocardial oxygen demand. In *Coronary Heart Disease Prevention, Detection, Rehabilitation with Emphasis on Exercise Testing.* ed. by S.M. Fox. Denver: International Medical Corp., 1974. pp. 219–221.

Boyer, J.: Effects of chronic exercise on cardiovascular function. Phys. Fitness Res. Digest, Series 2, i–5, 1972.

Bruce, R.A., et al.: Cardiac limitation to maximal oxygen transport and changes in components after jogging across the U.S. J. Appl. Physiol., *39*:958–963, 1975.

Bruce, R.A., Kusumi, F., and Hosmer, D.: Maximal oxygen intake and nomographic assessment of functional aerobic impairment in cardiovascular disease. Am. Heart J., *85*:546–562, 1973.

Brunner, D., and Meshulam, M.: Physical fitness of trained elderly people. In *Physical Activity and Aging.* Vol. 4 of *Medicine and Sport,* ed. by D. Brunner and E. Jokl. White Plains, N.Y.: A.J. Phiebig, 1969.

Burt, J., and Jackson, R.: The effects of physical exercise on the collateral circulation of dogs. J. Sports Med. Phys. Fitness, *5*:203–206, 1965.

Buskirk, E.R.: Cardiovascular adaptation to physical effort in healthy men. In *Exercise Testing and Exercise Training in Coronary Heart Disease.* ed. by J.P. Naughton and H.K. Hellerstein. New York: Academic Press, 1973, pp. 23–33.

Buskirk, E., and Taylor, H.L.: Maximal oxygen intake and its relation to body composition with special reference to chronic physical activity and obesity. J. Appl. Physiol., *11*:73, 1957.

Calculation of Metabolic Cost. Supplement to *Guidelines for Graded Exercise Testing and Exercise Prescription.* (On request.) American College of Sports Medicine, 1440 Monroe Street, 3002 Stadium, Madison, WI 53706

Cantwell, J.D.: Extreme bradycardia in middle-aged runners. Phys. Sports Med., *4*:55–57, 1976.

Carlson, L.A.: Lipid metabolism and muscular work. Fed. Proc., *26*:1755, 1967.

Carter, L., and Phillips, W.: Structural changes in exercising middle-aged males during a 2-year period. J. Appl. Physiol., *27*:787, 1969.

Choquette, G., and Ferguson, R.J.: Blood pressure reduction in "borderline" hypertensives following physical training. Can. Med. Assoc. J., *108*:699, 1973.

Clausen, J.P.: Effects of physical conditioning, a hypothesis concerning circulatory adjustment to exercise. (A review.) Scand. J. Clin. Lab. Invest., *24*:305, 1969.

Cohen, H., and Goldberg, C.: Effect of physical exercise on alimentary lipemia. Br. Med. J., *2*:509, 1960.

Cooper, K.H., et al.: Age-fitness adjusted maximal heart rates. In *The Role of Exercise in Internal Medicine,* Vol. 10 of *Medicine and Sport,* ed. by E. Jokl and D. Brunner. Basel: S. Karger AG, 1977. pp. 78–88.

Costill, D.L., Fink, W.J., and Pollock, M.L.: Muscle fiber composition and enzyme activities of elite distance runners. Med. Sci. Sports, *8*:96–100, 1976.

Crews, J., and Aldinger, E.: Effect of chronic exercise on myocardial function. Am. Heart J., *74*:536, 1967.

Cureton, T.: *The Physiological Effects of Exercise Program on Adults.* Springfield, Ill.: Charles C Thomas, 1971.

Currens, J.H., and White, P.D.: Half a century of running. New Engl. J. Med., *265*:988, 1961.

Damon, A., et al.: Predicting coronary heart disease from body measurements of Framingham males. J. Chronic Dis., *21*:781–802, 1969.

Daniel, B.J.: The effects of walking, jogging and running on the serum lipid concentration of the adult Caucasian male. Doctoral dissertation, University of So. Mississippi, 1969.

Dehn, M.M., and Bruce, R.A.: Longitudinal variations in maximal oxygen intake with age and activity. J. Appl. Physiol., *33*:805, 1972.

Denenberg, D.L.: The effects of exercise on the coronary collateral circulation. M.S. thesis, Boston University, 1969.

DeVilla, M., et al.: Correlation of quantitative submaximal exercise and ectopia with coronary arteriography and coronary collaterals. Circulation, *45–46(Suppl. II)*:II–145, 1972.

DeVries, H.: *Physiology of Exercise for Physical Education and Athletics.* Dubuque: Wm. C. Brown Co., 1974.

Doan, A.E., et al.: Myocardial ischemia after maximal exercise in healthy men. Am. Heart J., *69*:1, 1965.

Edington, D.W., and Cosmas, A.C.: Effect of maturation and training on mitochondrial size distributions in rat hearts. J. Appl. Physiol., *33*:715–725, 1972.

Ekblom, B., et al.: Effect of training on circulatory response to exercise. J. Appl. Physiol., *24*:518–528, 1968.

Erichsen, J.E.: The influence of the coronary circulation on the action of the heart. In *A Bibliography of Internal Medicine, Selected Diseases.* ed. by A.L. Bloomfield. Chicago: University of Chicago Press, 1960, pp. 18–19; London M. Gaz., *30*:561, 1842.

Falls, H., et al.: *Exercise Physiology.* New York: Academic Press, 1968.

Faris, A.W., Browning, F.M., and Ibach, J.D.: The effect of physical training upon total serum cholesterol levels and arterial distensibility of male white rats. J. Sports Med., *11*:24, 1971.

Ferguson, R.J., et al.: Effect of physical training on treadmill exercise capacity, collateral circulation and progression of coronary disease. Am. J. Cardiol., *34*:765, 1974.

Frick, M.H., Katila, M., and Sjogren, A.L.: Cardiac function and physical training after myocardial infarction. In *Coronary Heart Disease and Physical Fitness,* ed. by O.A. Larsen and R.O. Malmborg. Baltimore: University Park Press, 1971. p. 43.

Frick, M.H.: Coronary implications of hemodynamic changes caused by physical training. Am. J. Cardiol., *22*:417–425, 1968.

Frick, M.H., Konttinen, A., and Sarajas, H.S.S.: Effect of physical training on circulation at rest and during exercise. Am. J. Cardiol., *12*:142–147, 1963.

Fringer, M.N., and Stull, G.A.: Changes in cardiorespiratory parameters during periods of training and detraining in young females. Med. Sci. Sports, *6*:20–25, 1974.

Froelicher, V.: Animal studies of effect of chronic exercise on the heart and atherosclerosis. A review. Am. Heart J., *84*:496, 1972.

Froelicher, V.: The hemodynamic effects of physical conditioning in healthy, young, and middle-aged individuals, and in coronary heart disease patients. In *Exercise Testing and Exercise Training in Coronary Heart Disease.* ed. by J. Naughton and H. K. Hellerstein. New York: Academic Press, Inc. 1973. pp. 63–77.

Froelicher, V.: Prediction of maximal oxygen consumption. Chest, *68*:331–336, 1975.

Garcia-Palmieri, M.R., et al.: Interrelationship of serum lipids with relative weight, blood glucose, and physical activity. Circulation, *45*:829–836, 1972.

Geffen, L.B., et al.: Effects of exercise and physical fitness on human serum dopamine β-hydroxylase activity. Clin. Exp. Pharmac. Phys., *2*:35–38, 1975.

Glick, Z., and Kaufmann, N.A.: Weight and skinfold thickness changes during a physical training course. Med. Sci. Sports, *8(2)*:109–112, 1976.

Gollnick, P.D., Struck, P.J., and Bogyo, T.P.: Lactic dehydrogenase activities of rat heart and skeletal muscle after exercise and training. J. Appl. Physiol., *22*:623, 1967.

Gustafson, A.: Effect of training on blood lipids. In *Coronary Heart Disease and Physical Fitness.* ed. by A.O. Larsen and R.O. Malmborg. Baltimore: University Park Press, 1971. p. 126.

Gutin, B., Fogle, K., and Stewart, K.: Relationship among submaximal heart rate, aerobic power and running performance in children. Res. Qtr., *47(3)*:536–539, 1976.

Hall, V.E.: The relation of heart rate to exercise fitness: an attempt at physiological interpretation of the bradycardia of training. Pediatrics, *32*:723–729, 1963.

Hanson, J.S., et al.: Long term physical training and cardiovascular dynamics in middle-aged men. Circulation, *38*:783–799, 1968.

Hebert, J.A., and Lopez, A.: Metabolic effects of exercise. Residual metabolic effects of exercise in rats. Proc. Soc. Exp. Biol. Med., *148*:646, 1975.

Holloszy, J.: Effects of exercise on mitochondrial oxygen uptake and respiratory enzyme activity in skeletal muscle. J. Biol. Chem., *242*:2278, 1967.

Holloszy, J., et al.: Effect of six month training program of endurance exercise on serum lipids of middle-aged men. Am. J. Cardiol., *14*:753, 1964.

Ikkala, E., Myllyia, G., and Sarajas, H.S.S.: Platelet adhesiveness and adp-induced platelet aggregation in exercise. Ann. Med. Exp. Biol. Fenn., *44*:88–92, 1966.

Ira, G.H., Whalen, R.E., and Bogdonoff, M.D.: Heart rate changes in physicians during daily "stressful" tasks. J. Psychiatr. Res., *7*:147–150, 1963.

Jensen, C.R., and Fisher, A.G.: *Scientific Basis of Athletic Conditioning.* Philadelphia: Lea & Febiger, 1972.

Johnson, W., et al.: *Science and Medicine of Exercise and Sports.* New York: Harper & Row Publishers, 1960.

Kannel, W.B.: Some lessons in cardiovascular epidemiology from Framingham. Am. J. Cardiol., *37*:269–277, 1976.

Kannel, W.B., et al.: The relationship of adiposity to blood pressure and development of hypertension. Ann. Intern. Med., *57*:48–58, 1967.

Karvonen, M.J., and Barry, A.J.: *Physical Activity and the Heart.* Springfield, Ill.: Charles C Thomas, 1967.

Kasch, F. W.: The effects of exercise on the aging process. Phys. Sports Med., June, 1976, pp. 64–68.

Kasch, F.W.: The energy cost of walking and hiking. Phys. Sports Med., July, 1976, p. 49.

Katch, F.I., and Danielson, G.: Bicycle ergometer endurance in women related to maximal leg force, leg volume and body composition. Res. Qtr., *47(3)*:366–374, 1976.

Katz, L.N., and Feinberg, H.: The relation of cardiac effort to myocardial oxygen consumption and coronary flow. Circ. Res., *6*:656–669, 1958.

Kerr, A., Jr., Bommer, W.J., and Pilato, S.: Coronary artery enlargement in experimental cardiac hypertrophy. Am. Heart J., *75*:144, 1968.

Kilbom, A., et al.: Physical training in sedentary middle-aged and older men, Part I. Scand. J. Clin. Lab. Invest., *24*:315–322, 1969.

Kilbom, A.: Physical training in women. Scand. J. Clin. Lab. Invest., *28(Suppl. 19)*:1–34, 1971.

Kitamura, K., et al.: Hemodynamics correlates of myocardial oxygen consumption during upright exercise. J. Appl. Physiol., *32*:516–522, 1972.

Kiveloff, B., and Huber, O.: Brief maximal isometric exercise in hypertension. J. Amer. Geriatr. Soc., *19*:1006, 1971.

Kobernick, S.D., Niawayama, G., and Zuehlewski, A.C.: Effect of physical activity on cholesterol atherosclerosis in rabbits. Proc. Soc. Exp. Biol. Med., *96*:623, 1957.

Korge, P., and Viru, A.: Water and electrolyte metabolism in myocardium of exercising rats. J. Appl. Physiol., *31*:5–7, 1971.

Lamb, D.R., et al.: Glycogen, hexokinase, and glycogen synthetase adaptations to exercise. Am. J. Physiol., *217*:1628, 1969.

Langley, L.L., et al.: *Dynamic Anatomy and Physiology*. New York: McGraw-Hill, 1969.

Larson, L., et al.: *Encyclopedia of Sport, Sciences and Medicine*. New York: Macmillan Company, 1971.

Lellouch, J.: Blood pressure, morphology and obesity: relationship studied in a population of 1769 men. Rev. Epidem. Med. Soc. Sante Publique, *20*:185–194, 1972. (English Summary)

Leon, A., and Bloor, C.: Effects of exercise and its cessation on the heart and its blood supply. J. Appl. Physiol., *24*:485, 1968.

Leon, A., and Bloor, C.: Exercise effects on the heart at different ages. (Abstr.) Circulation, *41–42(Suppl. III)*:50, 1970.

Lersten, K.C.: *Physiology and Physical Conditioning*. Palo Alto: Peek Publications, 1971.

Lester, M., et al.: The effect of age and athletic training on the maximal heart rate during muscular exercise. Am. Heart J., *76*:370, 1968.

Lohman, F.W., et al.: Hypertension and myocardial infarction: behavior of blood pressure after infarction. Z. Kardiol., *63*:252–268, 1974. (English Summary)

Londeree, B. R., and Ames. S.A.: Trend analysis of the $\%VO_2$ max-HR regression. Med. Sci. Sports, *8(2)*:122–125, 1976.

Longhurst, J., Gifford, W., and Zelis, R.: Impaired forearm oxygen consumption during static exercise in patients with congestive heart failure. Circulation, *54(3)*:477–480, 1976.

Lown, B., et al.: Psychologic stress and threshold for repetitive ventricular response. Science, *182*:834, 1973.

MacDonald, G.A., and Fullerton, H.W.: Effects of physical activity on increased coagulation of blood after ingesting high-fat meal. Lancet, *2*:600, 1958.

Maddox, D.: Studying athletes to help the average man. Phys. Sports Med., *4*:113, 1976.

Magel, J.R., et al.: Specificity of swim training on maximum oxygen uptake. J. Appl. Physiol., *38*:151–155, 1974.

Massie, J.F., and Shephard, R.J.: Physiological and psychological effects of training. Med. Sci. Sports, *2*:1–6, 1970.

Mathew, D., and Fox, E.: *The Physiological Basis of Physical Education and Athletics*. Philadelphia: W. B. Saunders Company, 1971.

McConahay, D.R., et al.: Resting and exercise systolic time intervals. Circulation, *45*:592–601, 1972.

McCrimmon, D.R., et al.: Effect of training on plasma catecholamines in post myocardial infarction patients. Med. Sci. Sports, *8(3)*:152–156, 1976.

McDonough, J.R., et al.: Maximal cardiac output during exercise in patients with coronary artery disease. Am. J. Cardiol., *33*:23, 1974.

McHenry, P.L., et al.: Comparative study of exercise-induced ventricular arrhythmias in normal subjects and patients with documented coronary artery disease. Am. J. Cardiol., *37*:609–616, 1976.

Miller, M.A., and Leavell, L.C.: *Kimber-Gray-Stackpole's Anatomy and Physiology.* 16th ed. New York: Macmillan, 1972.

Mitchell, J.H., Sproule, B.J., and Chapman, C.V.: The physiological meaning of the maximal oxygen intake tests. J. Clin. Invest., *37*:538, 1958.

Montoye, H.J., et al.: Systolic pre-ejection period: patients with heart disease compared to normal subjects. Arch. Environ. Health, *21*:425–431, 1970.

Morris, J.N.: Epidemiology and cardiovascular disease of middle age. Mod. Concepts Cardiovasc. Dis., *29*:625, 1960.

Moxley, R.T., Brakman, P., and Astrup, T.: Resting levels of fibrinolysis in blood in inactive and exercising men. J. Appl. Physiol., *28*:549, 1970.

National Center for Health Statistics: Chronic conditions and limitations of activity and mobility. U.S. July, 1965–June, 1967. U.S. Health Service, Series 10, No. 61, 1971.

Naughton, J., Balke, B., and Nagle, F.: Refinements in methods of evaluation and physical conditioning before and after myocardial infarction. Am. J. Cardiol., *14*: 837, 1964.

Nemec, E.D., Mansfield, L., and Kennedy, J.W.: Heart rate and blood pressure responses during sexual activity in normal males. Am. Heart J., *92(3)*:274–277, 1976.

Nestel, P.J., et al.: Catecholamine secretion and sympathetic nervous responses to emotion in men with and without angina pectoris. Am. Heart J., *73*: 227–234, 1967.

Niederberger, M., et al.: Disparities in ventilatory and circulatory responses to bicycle and treadmill exercise. Br. Heart J., *36*:377–382, 1974.

Nikkila, E.K.: Effect of physical activity on post-prandial levels of fat in the serum. Lancet, *1*:1151, 1962.

Nowlin, J.B., et al.: The association of nocturnal angina pectoris with dreaming. Ann. Intern. Med., *63*:1040, 1965.

Nutter, D.O., Schlant, R.C., and Hurst, J.W.: Isometric exercise and the cardiovascular system. Med. Concepts Cardiovasc. Dis., *41*:11–15, 1972.

Oakes, T.W., et al.: Social factors in newly discovered elevated blood pressure. J. Health Soc. Behav., *14*:198–204, 1973.

Oliver, R.M.: Physique and serum lipids of young London busmen in relation to ischemic heart disease. Br. J. Ind. Med., *24*:181–187, 1967.

Oscai, L.B., et al.: Cardiac growth and respiratory enzyme levels in male rats subjected to a running program. Am. J. Physiol., *220*:1238, 1971.

Oscai, L.B., Mole, P.A., and Holloszy, J.O.: Effects of exercise on cardiac weight and mitochondria in male and female rats. Am. J. Physiol., *220*:1944, 1971.

Oscai, L.B., et al.: Normalization of serum triglycerides and lipoprotein elec-
    trophoretic patterns by exercise. Abstr. 19th Annual meeting, American
    College of Sports Medicine, May 1–3, 1972.
Penpargkul, S., and Scheuer, J.: The effect of physical training upon the mechanical
    and metabolic performance of the rat heart. J. Clin. Invest., 49:1859, 1970.
Pernow, B., and Saltin, B.: *Muscle Metabolism during Exercise: Advances in
    Experimental Medicine and Biology.* Vol. 2. New York: Plenum Press, 1971.
Poland, J.L., and Blount, D.H.: The effects of training on myocardial metabolism.
    Proc. Soc. Exp. Biol. Med., 129:177, 1968.
Pollock, M.J., et al.: Effects of frequency of training on serum lipids, cardiovascular
    function and body composition. In *Exercise and Fitness,* ed. by B. Don
    Franks. Chicago: Chicago Athletic Institute, 1969, p. 161.
Pollock, M.L., et al.: Effect of training two days per week at different intensities on
    middle-aged men. Med. Sci. Sports, 4:192–197, 1974.
Poupa, O.K., Rakusan, K., and Ostadal, B.: The effect of physical activity upon the
    heart of vertebrates. In *Physical Activity and Aging.* Vol. 4 of *Medicine and
    Sport,* ed. by D. Brunner and E. Jokl. White Plains, N.Y.: A.J. Phiebig, 1969.
Raskoff, Wm. J., Goldman, S., and Cohn, K.: The "athletic heart." JAMA,
    236(2):158–162, 1976.
Ricci, B.: *Experiments in the Physiology of Human Performance.* Philadelphia: Lea
    & Febiger, 1970.
Ricci, B.: *Physical and Physiological Conditioning for Men.* Dubuque, Ia.: Wm. C.
    Brown Publishers, 1966.
Roeske, Wm., et al.: Noninvasive evaluation of ventricular hypertrophy in profes-
    sional athletes. Circulation, 53(2):286–292, 1976.
Rosing, D.R., et al.: Blood fibrinolytic activity in man: diurnal variation and the
    response to varying intensities of exercise. Circ. Res., 27:171, 1970.
Roskamm, H.: Optimum patterns of exercise for healthy adults. Can. Med. Assoc.
    J., 96:895, 1967.
Roskamm, H.: General circulatory adjustment to exercise in well trained subjects. In
    Coronary Heart Disease and Physical Fitness. ed. by O.A. Larsen and R.O.
    Malmborg. Baltimore: University Park Press, 1971. pp. 17–20.
Ross, R., and Glomset, A.: Atherosclerosis and the arterial smooth muscle cell.
    Science, 180:1332–1339, 1973.
Rowe, D.G., et al.: Effects of different intensities of exercise on intraocular pressure.
    Res. Qtr., 47(3):436–444, 1976.
Ryan, A.J.: Carotid palpation practice questioned. Phys. Sports Med., Sept., 1976,
    p. 23.
Saltin, B., et al.: Response to exercise after bed rest and after training. Circulation,
    48(Suppl. VII):1–55, 1968.
Sannerstedt, R.: Hemodynamic findings at rest and during exercise in mild arterial
    hypertension. Am. J. Med. Science, 258:70–79, 1959.
Schaper, W.: Pathophysiology of coronary circulation. Prog. Cardiovasc. Dis.,
    14:275–296, 1971.
Scheuer, J., and Stezoski, S.W.: Effect of physical training on the mechanical and
    metabolic response of the rat heart to hypoxia. Circ. Res., 30:418, 1972.
Scheuer, J., Kapner, L., and Stringfellow, C.: Glycogen, lipid, and high energy,
    phosphate stores in hearts from conditioned rats. J. Lab. Clin. Med., 75:924–
    929, 1970.

Shane, S.: Relationship between serum lipids and physical conditioning. Am. J. Cardiol., *18*:540, 1966.

Sharkey, B.J.: *Physiology and Physical Activity.* New York: Harper and Row, 1975.

Sheehan, G.: Measuring maximums on a merciless machine. Phys. Sports Med., Sept., 1976, p. 38.

Shennum, P.L., and DeVries, H.: The effect of saddle height on oxygen consumption during bicycle ergometer work. Med. Sci. Sports, *8(2)*:119–121, 1976.

Shephard, R.J.: *Endurance Fitness.* Toronto: University of Toronto Press, 1969.

Simon, L.M., Scheuer, J., and Robin, E.D.: Cytochrome oxidase and pyruvate kinase changes in the chronically exercised rats. (Abstr.) Clin. Res., *19*:340, 1971.

Simpson, M.T., et al.: An epidemiological study of platelet aggregation and physical activity. (Abstr.) Circulation, *43–44(Suppl)*:11–88, 1971.

Snyder, F., et al.: Changes in respiration, heart rate and systolic blood pressure in human sleep. J. Appl. Physiol., *19*:417, 1964.

Stevenson, J.A.F., et al.: Effect of exercise on coronary tree size in rats. Circ. Res., *15*:265, 1964.

Tabakin, B.S., Hanson, J.S., and Levy, A.M.: Effects of physical training on the cardiovascular and respiratory response to graded upright exercise in distance runners. Br. Heart J., *27*:205–210, 1965.

Tomanek, R.J.: Effects of age and exercise on the extent of the myocardial capillary bed. Anat. Rec., *167*:55, 1970.

Tomanek, R.J., Taunton, C.A., and Liskop, K.S.: Relationship between age, chronic exercise and connective tissue of the heart. J. Gerontol., *27*:33, 1972.

Vander, A.J., Sherman, J.H., and Luciano, D.: *Human Physiology.* 2nd ed. New York: McGraw-Hill, 1975.

Vlodaver, Z., and Edwards, J.E.: Pathology of coronary atherosclerosis. Prog. Cardiovasc. Dis., *14*:256–274, 1971.

Warnoch, N.H., et al.: Effects of exercise on blood coagulation time and atherosclerosis of cholesterol-fed cockerels. Circ. Res., *5*:478, 1957.

Weltman, A., and Katch, V.: Min-by-min respiratory exchange and oxygen uptake kinetics during steady-state exercise in subjects of high and low Max VO_2. Res. Qtr., *47(3)*:490–498, 1976.

Wilkerson, J.E., Evonuk, E.: Changes in cardiac and skeletal muscle myosin ATPase activities after exercise. J. Appl. Physiol., *30*:328, 1971.

Williams, L.R.T.: Work output and heart rate response of top level New Zealand oarsmen. Res. Qtr., *47(3)*:506–512, 1976.

Wilmore, J.: *Exercise and Sport Sciences Reviews.* Vols. I, II, III. New York: Academic Press, 1973, 1974, 1975.

Wilmore, J.: et al.: Football pros' and strengths—and cv weakness—charted. *Phys. Sports Med.,* Oct., 1976, pp. 45–54

EXERCISE TESTING AND EXERCISE PRESCRIPTION

American College of Sports Medicine: *Guidelines for Graded Exercise Testing and Exercise Prescription.* Philadelphia: Lea & Febiger, 1975.

Aronow, W.S., and Cassidy, J.: Five year follow-up of double Master's test, maximal treadmill stress test, and resting and postexercise apexcardiogram in asymptomatic persons. Circulation, *52*:616–618, 1975.

Aronow, W.S.: Thirty-month follow-up of maximal treadmill stress test and double Master's test in normal subjects. Circulation, 47:287–292, 1973.

Ascoop, C.A., et al.: Exercise test, history and serum lipid levels in patients with chest pain and normal electrocardiogram at rest: comparison to findings at coronary arteriography. Am. Heart J., 82:609–617, 1971.

Bartel, A.G., et al.: Graded exercise stress tests in angiographically documented coronary artery disease. Circulation, 49:348–356, 1974.

Bellet, S., and Roman, L.: Comparison of the double two-step test and the maximal exercise treadmill test. Circulation, 36:238, 1957.

Bellet, S., et al.: Detection of coronary-prone subjects in a normal population by radioelectrocardiographic exercise test: follow-up studies. Am. J. Cardiol., 19:783–787, 1967.

Blorck, G.: Early diagnosis of coronary heart disease. Adv. Cardiol., 8:25–37, 1973.

Blomqvist, C.G., and Atkins, J.M.: Repeated exercise testing in patients with angina pectoris: reproducibility and follow-up results. Circulation, 44(Suppl. II):II-76, 1971.

Blomqvist, C.G.: Use of exercise testing for diagnostic and functional evaluation of patients with arteriosclerotic heart disease. Circulation, 44:1120–1136, 1971.

Borer, J.S., et al.: Limitations of the electrocardiographic response to exercise in predicting coronary artery disease. N. Engl. J. Med., 293:367–372, 1975.

Bruce, R.A.: Atherosclerosis. in Coronary Heart Disease Prevention, Detection, Rehabilitation with Emphasis on Exercise Testing. ed. by S. Fox. Denver: International Medical Corp., 1974, pp. 5–11.

Bruce, R.A., and Hornsten, T.R.: Exercise stress testing in evaluation of patients with ischemic heart disease. Prog. Cardiovasc. Dis., 11:371–390, 1969.

Bruce, R.A.: Exercise testing of patients with coronary heart disease. Ann. Clin. Res., 3:323–332, 1971.

Bruce, R.A., et al.: Exercising testing in adult normal subjects and cardiac patients. Pediatrics, 32:742–756, 1963.

Bruce, R.A., and McDonough, J.R.: Stress testing in screening for cardiovascular disease. Bull. N.Y. Acad. Med., 45:1288–1295, 1969.

Bruce, R.A., et al.: Quantitation of QRS and ST-segment responses to exercise. Am. Heart J., 71:455, 1966.

Bruce, R.A.: Values and limitations of exercise electrocardiography. Circulation, 50:1–4, 1974.

Cantwell, J., and Fletcher, G.: Exercise and Coronary Heart Disease. Springfield, Ill.: Charles C Thomas, 1975.

Cissik, J.H., Salustro, J., and Patton, O.L.: Pulmonary exercise stress testing: a discussion. J. Cardiovasc. Pulmon. Technol., May/June, 1976, pp. 33–37.

Cohn, P.F., et al.: Diagnostic accuracy of two-step post exercise ECG. Results in 305 subjects studied by coronary arteriography. JAMA, 220:501, 1972.

Committee on Exercise and Physical Fitness of the AMA and President's Council on Physical Fitness and Sports: Evaluation for exercise participation. JAMA, 219(7):900–901, 1972.

Cooksey, J.D., Parker, B.M., and Bahl, O.P.: The diagnostic contribution of exercise testing in left bundle branch block. Am. Heart J., 88:482–486, 1974.

Cooper, K.H.: The treadmill test for heart disease. Business Week, Jan., 1974, pp. 70–71.

Cumming, G.R., et al.: Electrocardiographic changes during exercise in asymptomatic men; 3-year follow-up. Can. Med. Assoc. J., *112*:578–581, 1975.

Cumming, G.R.: Yield of ischemic exercise electrocardiograms in relation to exercise intensity in a normal population. Br. Heart J., *34*:919–923, 1972.

Demany, M.A., Tambe, A., and Zimmerman, H.A.: Correlation between coronary arteriography and the post-exercise electrocardiogram. Am. J. Cardiol., *19*:526, 1967.

Detry, J.R.: *Exercise Testing and Training in Coronary Heart Disease.* Baltimore: Williams & Wilkins Company, 1973.

Doyle, J.T., and Kinch, S.H.: The prognosis of an abnormal electrocardiographic stress test. Circulation, *41*:545, 1970.

Ellestad, M.H., et al.: Maximal treadmill stress testing for cardiovascular evaluation. Circulation, *39*:517–522, 1969.

Ellestad, M.H., and Wan, M.K.C.: Predictive implications of stress testing. Circulation, *51*:363–369, 1975.

Ellestad, M.: *Stress Testing: Principles and Practice.* Philadelphia: F. A. Davis Publishers, 1975.

Ellestad, M., McHenry, P.L., and Froelicher, V.F.: Stress testing: how valuable is it in asymptomatic CAD population? Clin. Trends Cardiol., *5(5)*, May-June, 1976.

Epstein, S.E.: Exercise stress testing held overused in CAD diagnosis; lack of sensitivity cited. Clin. Trends Cardiol., *2(4)*, April-May, 1973.

Erikssen, J., et al.: False positive diagnostic tests and coronary angiographic findings in 105 presumably healthy males. Circulation, *54(3)*:371–376, 1976.

Exercise Testing and Training of Apparently Healthy Individuals: A Handbook for Physicians. American Heart Association, 1972.

Exercise Testing and Training of Individuals with Heart Disease or at High Risk for its Development: A Handbook for Physicians. American Heart Association, 1975.

Faris, J.V., et al.; Prevalence and reproducibility of exercise-induced ventricular arrhythmias during maximal exercise testing in normal men. Am. J. Cardiol., *37*:617–622, 1976.

Fitzgibbon, G.M., et al.: A double Master's two step test: clinical, angiographic and hemodynamic correlations. Ann. Intern. Med., *74*:509, 1971.

Fox, S., et al.: *Coronary Heart Disease: Prevention, Detection, Rehabilitation with Emphasis on Exercise Testing.* Denver: International Medical Corporation, 1974.

Froelicher, V.F.: The application of electrocardiographic screening and exercise testing to preventive cardiology. Prev. Med., *2*:592–599, 1973.

Froelicher, V.F., et al.: Epidemiologic study of asymptomatic men screened by maximal treadmill testing for latent coronary arrtery disease. Am. J. Cardiol., *34*:770, 1974.

Froelicher, V.F., et al.: The value of exercise testing for screening asymptomatic men for latent coronary artery disease. Prog. Cardiovasc. Dis., *18*:265–272, 1976.

Harris, C., et al.: Treadmill stress test in left ventricular hypertrophy. Chest, *63*:353–357, 1973.

Hellerstein, H.K.: Exercise tests inadequate for cardiac patients. Phys. Sports Med., 4:58–62, 1976.

Hellerstein, H.K., et al.: Principles of exercise prescription. In *Exercise Testing and Exercise Training in Coronary Heart Disease*. ed. by J.P. Naughton and H.K. Hellerstein. New York: Academic Press, 1973, pp. 29–167.

Hellerstein, H., et al.: Two-step exercise test as a test of cardiac function and chronic rheumatic heart disease and arteriosclerotic heart disease with old myocardial infarction. Am. J. Cardiol., 7:234–242, 1961.

Inagaki, Y.: Effects of treadmill exercise on the timing of the heart and arterial sounds and the slope of the brachial arterial pulse wave. Am. Heart J., 92(3):282–289, 1976.

Jenkins, C.D., Rosenman, R.H., and Friedman, M.: Development of an objective psychological test for the determination of the coronary prone behavior pattern in employed men. J. Chronic. Dis., 20:371–379, 1967.

Kaplan, M.A., et al.: Inability of the submaximal treadmill stress test to predict the location of coronary disease. Circulation, 47:250, 1973.

Kasselbaum, D.G., Sutherland, K.I., and Judkins, M.P.: A comparison of hypoxemia and exercise electrocardiography in CAD. Am. Heart J., 75:759–774, 1969.

Kattus, A.A.: Exercise electrocardiography: recognition of the ischemic response, false positive and negative patterns. Am. J. Cardiol., 33:721–731, 1974.

Kattus, A.A.: Exercise testing and therapy in ischemic heart disease. J. S.C. Med. Assoc., 65:57–60, 1969.

Kattus, A.A., and MacAlpin, R.N.: Role of exercise in discovery, evaluation, and management of ischemic heart disease. In *Cardiovascular Clinics: Coronary Heart Disease*, ed. by A. Brest. Philadelphia: F.A. Davis Co., 1969, pp. 255–279.

Kattus, A.A., Alvaro, A., and MacAlpin, R.N.: Treadmill tests for capacity and adaptation in angina pectoris. J. Occup. Med., 10:627, 1968.

Kattus, A.A.: S-T segment depression with near maximal exercise: its modification by physical conditioning. Chest, 62:678–683, 1972.

Kavanagh, T.: Postcoronary joggers need precise guidelines. Phys. Sports Med., 4:63–65, 1976.

Keleman, M.H., et al.: Diagnosis of obstructive coronary disease by maximal exercise and atrial pacing. Circulation, 48:1227–1233, 1973.

Kemp, G.L.: Electrocardiogram abnormalities discovered with treadmill stress testing. Heart and Lung, 2:227–231, 1973.

Kemp, G.L.: Value of treadmill stress testing in variant angina pectoris. Am. J. Cardiol., 30:781–783, 1972.

Lapin, E.S., et al.: Changes in maximal exercise performance in the evaluation of saphenous vein bypass surgery. Circulation, 47:1164, 1973.

Larsen, O., and Malmborg, R. (eds.): *Coronary Heart Disease and Physical Fitness*. Baltimore: University Park Press, 1971.

Levenson, R.: Role of exercise test in evaluation of cardiac patients. JAMA, 183:480, 1963.

McDonough, J.F., and Bruce, R.A.: Maximal exercise testing in assessing C.V. function. J. S.C. Med. Assoc., 65:18–33, 1959.

Master, A.M.: Exercise and stress testing, the Master two-step test; some historical highlights and current concepts. J. S.C. Med. Assoc., *65(Suppl. 12)*:12–17, 1969.

McHenry, P.L., Phillips, J.F., and Knoebel, S.B.: Correlation of computer quantitated treadmill exercise electrocardiogram with arteriographic location of coronary artery disease. Am. J. Cardiol., *30*:747–752, 1972.

Morse, R., et al.: *Exercise and the Heart: Guidelines for Exercise Programs.* Springfield, Ill.: Charles C Thomas Publishers, 1972.

Naughton, J., Patterson, J., and Fox, S.M.: Exercise tests in patients with chronic disease. J. Chronic Dis., *24*:519–522, 1971.

Naughton, J., et al.: *Exercise Testing and Exercise Training in Coronary Heart Disease.* New York: Academic Press, 1973.

Office evaluation of physical finess. Phys. Sports Med., June, 1976, pp. 81–93.

Pollock, M.L., et al.: A comparative analysis of four protocols for maximal treadmill stress testing. Am. Heart J., *92*:39–46, 1976..

Redwood, D.R., et al.: Importance of the design of an exercise protocol in the evaluations of patients with angina pectoris. Circulation, *43*:618, 1971.

Redwood, D.R., and Epstein, S.E.: Uses and limitations of stress testing in the evaluation of ischemic heart disease. Circulation, *46*:1115, 1972.

Reedy, C.: Introduction. In *Exercise Testing and Exercise Training in Coronary Heart Disease,* ed. by J.P. Naughton, H.K. Hellerstein, et al. New York: Academic Press, 1973. pp. xvii–xx.

Riley, C.P., et al.: Submaximal exercise testing in a roundup sample of an elderly population. Circulation, *42*:43, 1970.

Rochmis, P., and Blackburn, H.: Exercise tests: a survey of procedures, safety and litigation experience in approximately 170,000 tests. JAMA, *217*:1061–1066, 1971.

Roitman, D., Jones, W.B., and Sheffield, L.T.: Comparison of submaximal exercise ECG test with coronary cineangiocardiogram. Ann. Intern. Med., *72*:641–647, 1970.

Schmidt, C.: Stress testing: theory vs. practice. J. Cardiovasc. Pulmon. Technol., *1*:15, July-Aug., 1973.

Sharrock, N., Garrett, H.L., and Mann, G.V.: Practical exercise test for physical fitness and cardiac performance. Am. J. Cardiol., *30*:727–732, 1972.

Sheffield, L.T., Holt, J.H., and Reeves, T.J.: Exercise graded by heart rate in electrocardiographic testing for angina pectoris. Circulation, *32*:622, 1965.

Sheffield, L.T., and Reeves, T.J.: Graded exercise in the diagnosis of angina pectoris. Mod. Concepts Cardiovasc. Dis., *34*:1, 1965.

Sheffield, L.T., Roitman, D., and Reeves, T.J.: Submaximal exercise testing. J. S.Car. Med. Assoc., *65*:18–25, 1969.

Sketch, M.H., et al.: Sex differences in stress testing. Am. J. Cardiol., *38*:135–137, 1976.

Smokler, E.P., et al.: Reproducibility of multistage near maximal treadmill test for exercise tolerance in angina pectoris. Circulation, *48*:346, 1973.

Spangler, R.D., et al.: A submaximal exercise electrocardiographic test as a method of detecting occult ischemic heart disease. Am. Heart J., *80*:752–758, 1970.

Spodick, D.H., and Lance, V.Q.: Noninvasive stress testing. Circulation, *53(4)*:673–676, 1976.

Stoedefalke, K.G.: The principles of conducting exercise programs. In *Exercise Testing and Exercise Training in Coronary Heart Disease*. ed. by Naughton, J., et al. New York: Academic Press, 1973. pp. 299–305.

Vecchio, T.J.: Predictive value of a single diagnostic test in unselected population. N. Engl. J. Med., *274*:1171–74, 1966.

Wilson, P.K. (ed.): *Adult Fitness and Cardiac Rehabilitation*. Baltimore: University Park Press, 1975.

Wilson, P.K., Karatun, O., and Edgett, J.W.: Basics of graded exercise testing. J. Cardiovasc. Pulmon. Technol., *3(4)*:17, 1975.

Wilson, P.K., and Gushiken, T.T.: Exercise testing and exercise therapy. *American Physical Therapy Association*, Newsletter, Vol. 2, No. 1, April, 1976.

Zohman, L., et al.: *Medical Aspects of Exercise Testing and Training*. New York: Intercontinental Medical Book Corporation, 1973.

FUNCTIONAL ANATOMY

Crouch, J.E.: *Functional Human Anatomy*, 3rd ed. Philadelphia: Lea & Febiger, 1978.

Goss, C.M. (ed.): *Gray's Anatomy of the Human Body*. 29th American edition. Philadelphia: Lea & Febiger, 1973.

Haber, L.D.: The epidemiology of disability. The measurement of functional capacity limitations. Social Security Survey of the Disabled: 1966. Report No. 10, Washington, D.C., 1970.

Heyden, S.: Epidemiology. In *Arteriosclerosis*. ed. by F.G. Schettler and G.S. Boyd. Amsterdam: Elsevier Publishing Co., 1969. p. 266

Houte, O.V., and Kesteloot, H.: An epidemiological survey of risk factors for ischemic H.D. in 42804 men, I. Serum cholesterol value. Acta Cardiol. (Brux.), *27*:527–564, 1972.

Kiesling, H.K., Piehl, K., and Lundqvist, C.G.: The number and size of skeletal muscle mitochondria. In *Coronary Heart Disease and Physical Fitness*, ed. by O.A. Larsen and R.O. Malmborg. Baltimore: University Park Press, 1971, pp. 143–146.

Linzbach, A.J.: Heart failure from the point of view of quantitative anatomy. Am. J. Cardiol., *5*:370, 1960.

National Institute of Health: *National Heart, Blood Vessel, Lung and Blood Program Report*. U.S. Dept. of HEW: Public Health Service Publications, Vol. 4, 1973.

Netter, F.H., and Yonkman, F.F.: *The CIBA Collection of Medical Illustrations*. Vol. 5, Heart. New York: Ciba Publications, 1969. pp. 210–214.

Morris, J.N., Heady, J.A., and Raffle, P.A.: Physique of London busmen: epidemiology of uniforms. Lancet, *2*:569–570, 1956.

Pansky, B., and House, E.L.: *Review of Gross Anatomy*. ed. 2. New York: Macmillan, 1969.

Rasch, P., and Burke, R.: *Kinesiology and Applied Anatomy*. 5th ed. Philadelphia: Lea & Febiger, 1974.

Thompson, C.: *Manual of Structural Kinesiology*. St. Louis: C.V. Mosby, 1969.

Wilson, P.K., Floyd, W.A., and Culver, A.B.: *Human Anatomy and Physiology of the Muscular, Nervous, Skeletal, Reproductive Systems, and Body Tissues*, 2nd ed. Dubuque: Kendall-Hunt Publishing Co., 1973.

HEART DISEASE

Acheson, R.: The etiology of coronary heart disease. Yale J. Biol. Med., *35*:143–170, 1962.

Amsterdam, E.A., and Ebert, P.A.: Angina pectoris: two perspectives. Clin. Trends Cardiol., *5(6)*, 1976.

Banister, E.W., and Taunton, J.E.: A rehabilitation program after myocardial infarction. Br. Columbia Med. J., *13*:233–235, 1971.

Bassler, T.J.: Take heart. In Reader's Comments of *Runner's World Magazine*, Sept., 1976, p. 84.

Bellett, S., et al.: Continuous electrocardiographic monitoring during automobile driving. Studies in normal subjects and patients with coronary disease. Am. J. Cardiol., *22*:856, 1968.

Breslow, L., and Buell, P.: Mortality from coronary heart disease and physical activity of work in California. J. Chronic Dis., *11*:421, 1960.

Bruce, R.A., and Kluge, W.: Defibrillatory treatment of exertional cardiac arrest in coronary disease. JAMA, *216*:653, 1971.

Bruhn, J.G., McCrady, K.E., and DuPlessis, A.: Evidence of emotional drain preceding death from myocardial infarction. Psychiat. Dig., *29*:34, 1968.

Bruhn, J.G., et al.: Social aspects of coronary heart disease in a Pennsylvania German community. Soc. Sci. Med., *2*:201, 1968.

Cairns, J.A., Fantus, I., and Klassen, G.: Unstable angina pectoris. Am. Heart J., *92(3)*:373–386, 1976.

Cassem, N.H., and Hackett, T.P.: Psychological rehabilitation of MI patients in the acute phase. Heart and Lung, *2*:382, 1973.

Chiang, B.N., et al.: Relationship of premature systoles to coronary heart disease and sudden death in the Tecumseh epidemiologic study. Ann. Intern. Med., *70*:1159–1166, 1969.

Clark, D.A., Allen, M.F., and Wilson, F.H., Jr.: USAFSAM cardiovascular disease follow-up study, 1972 progress report. Aerospace Med., *43*:194–197, 1973.

Cohen, L.S., Elliott, W.C., and Gorlin, R.: Coronary heart disease: clinical, cinearteriographic and metabolic correlations. Am. J. Cardiol., *17*:153, 1966.

Cook, L.P.: The coronary spectrum. Statistics, magnitude of the problem. J. Rehab., *32*:17–18, 1966.

Croog, S.H., and Levine, S.: Social status and subjective perceptions of 250 men after myocardial infarction. Public Health Rep., *84*:989, 1969.

Dishart, M.: A national study of 84,699 applicants for services from State vocational rehabilitation agencies in the United States. Washington, D.C., National Rehabilitation Assoc., 1964.

Eckstein, R.W.: Effect of exercise and coronary artery narrowing on cholesterol circulation. Circ. Res., *5*:230–234, 1957.

Eliot, R.S., Baroldi, G., and Leone, A.: Necropsy studies in myocardial infarction with minimal or no coronary luminal reduction due to atherosclerosis. Circulation, *49*:1127–1132, 1974.

Enos, W.F., Holmes, R.H., and Beyer, J.: Coronary disease among U.S. soldiers killed in action in Korea. JAMA, *152*:1090–1093, 1953.

Epstein, S.E., et al.: Angina pectoris: pathophysiology, evaluation and treatment. Ann. Intern. Med., *75*:263–296, 1971.

Eugene, S.L., et al.: Changes in maximum exercise performance in the evaluation of saphenous vein bypass surgery. Circulation, *57*:1164–1173, 1973.

Forssman, O., and Lindegard, B.: The post-coronary patient. A multidisciplinary investigation of middle-aged Swedish males. J. Psychosom. Res., *3*:89, 1958.

Frank, C.W., Weinblatt, E., and Shapiro, S.: Prognostic implications of serum cholesterol in coronary heart disease. In *Atherosclerosis: Proceedings Second International Symposium,* ed. by R.J. Jones. New York: Springer-Verlag, 1970, pp. 390–398.

Friedberg, C.K.: *Diseases of the Heart.* Philadelphia: W.B. Saunders, 1969.

Fulmer, H.S., and Roberts, R.W.: Coronary heart disease among the Navajo Indians. Ann. Intern. Med., *59*:740–764, 1963.

Fulton, M.D., et al.: Sudden death and myocardial infarction. Circulation, *40(Suppl. IV)*:IV-182, IV-191, 1969.

Goldstein, S., et al.: Sudden death in acute myocardial infarction. Arch. Intern. Med., *129*:720, 1972.

Goodwin, J.F., and Oakley, C.M.: The cardiomyopathies. In Jones (ed.) *Modern Trends in Cardiology,* 2nd Series, ed. by A.M. Jones. New York: Appleton-Century-Crofts, 1969, pp. 256–292.

Gordon, T., and Kannel, W.B.: Predisposition to atherosclerosis in the head, heart and legs, the Framingham study. JAMA, *221*:671, 1972.

Gorlin, R.: *Coronary Heart Disease.* Morris Plains, N.J.: Warner-Chilcott Laboratories, 1972, p. 7.

Green, L.H.: Fatal myocardial infarction in marathon racing. Ann. Intern. Med., *84*:704–706, 1976.

Haber. L.D.: The disabled worker under OASDI. Washington, D.C.: U.S. Dept. of HEW, Division of Research and Statistics, Research Report, 1964.

Hamburger, W.W.: The earliest known reference to the heart and circulation, the Edwin Smith surgical papyrus, circa 3000 B.C. Am. Heart J., *17*:259, 1939.

Hayes, M.J., Morris, G.K., and Hampton, J.R.: Comparison of mobilization after two and nine days in incompleted myocardial infarction. Br. Med. J., *3*:10–13, 1974.

Hellerstein, H.K., and Friedman, E.H.: Sexual activity and the post-coronary patient. Arch. Intern. Med., *125*:987, 1970.

Herrick, J.B.: Thrombosis of the coronary arteries. JAMA, *72*:387, 1919.

Herrick, J.B.: Clinical features of sudden obstruction of the coronary arteries. JAMA, *59*:2015, 1912.

Hinkle, L.E., Jr., et al.: Studies in ecology of coronary heart disease. Variations in the human electrocardiogram under conditions of daily life. Arch. Environ. Health, *9*:14, July, 1964.

Hinkle, L.E.: CHD and sudden death in actively employed American men. Bull. N.Y. Acad. Med., *49*:467–474, 1973.

Holmgren, A.: Vasoregulatory asthenia. In *Coronary Heart Disease and Physical Fitness,* ed. by O.A. Larsen, and R.O. Malmborg. Baltimore: University Park Press, 1971. pp. 34–37.

Hultgren, H., et al.: A clinical evaluation of coronary arteriography. Am. J. Med., *42*:228, 1967.

Intersociety Commission for Heart Disease: Primary prevention of the atherosclerotic diseases. Circulation, *42*:A-55–67, 1970.

Jenkins, C.D., et al.: Association of coronary prone behavior scores with recurrence of coronary heart disease. J. Chronic Dis., *24*:601, 1971.

Kagan, A., Dawber, T.R., Kannel, W.B., and Revotskie, N.: The Framingham study: a prospective study of coronary heart disease. Fed. Proc., *21*:52–57, 1962.

Kahn, H.A.: The relationship of reported coronary heart disease mortality to physical activity of work. Am. J. Public Health, *53*:1058, 1963.

Kannel, W.B., and Gordon, T.: Premature mortality for coronary heart disease, the Framingham study. JAMA, *215*:1617–1625, 1971.

Kannel, W.B., Castelli, W.P., and McNamara, P.M.: The coronary profile: 12 year follow up in the Framingham study. J. Occup. Med., *9*:611–619, 1967.

Keys, A.: Coronary heart disease—the global picture. Atherosclerosis, *22*:149–192, 1975.

Keys, A., et al.: Mortality and coronary heart disease among men studied for 23 years. Arch. Intern. Med., *128*:201–214, 1971.

Keys, A.: Concluding remarks. In *Atherosclerosis: Proceedings Second International Symposium*. ed. by R.J. Jones. New York: Springer-Verlag, 1970. pp. 399–405.

Khan, A.H., and Haywood, L.J.: Myocardial infarction in nine patients with radiologically patent coronary arteries. N. Engl. J. Med., *291*:427–431, 1974.

Klein, R.F., et al.: Transfer from a CCU. Some adverse response. Arch. Intern. Med., *122*:104, 1968.

Lavine, P., et al.: Left main coronary artery disease. Am. J. Cardiol., *30*:791, 1972.

Lee, K.T., et al.: Geographic studies of arteriosclerosis. Arch. Environ. Health, *4*:4–10, 1962.

Lenard, H.: Issues for the rehabilitation counselor. J. Rehabil., *24*:12, 1963.

Levy, R.I., and Stone, N.J.: The metabolic basis and management of inherited premature ischemic heart disease. In *Changing Concepts in Cardiovascular Disease*. ed. by H.I. Russek and B.L. Zohman. Baltimore: Williams and Wilkins, 1972. pp. 32–39.

Mallory, G.K., White, P.D., and Salgar, S.J.: The speed of healing of myocardial infarction. Am. Heart J., *18*:647, 1939.

Maseri, A., Mimmo, R., and Chierchia, S.: Coronary artery spasm as a cause of acute myocardial ischemia in man. Chest, *68*:625–629, 1975.

McDonough, J.R., et al.: Coronary heart disease among negroes and whites in Evans County, Georgia. J. Chronic Dis., *18*:443–468, 1968.

McNamara, S.S., et al.: Coronary artery disease in combat casualties in Vietnam. JAMA, *216*:1185–1187, 1971.

Mead, W.F., et al.: Successful resuscitation of two near simultaneous cases of cardiac arrest with a review of fifteen cases occurring during supervised exercise. Circulation, *53(1)*:187–189, 1976.

Miall, W.E., et al.: Longitudinal study of heart disease in a Jamaican rural population: factors influencing mortality. Bull. WHO, *46*:685–694, 1972.

Mitrani, Y., Karplus, H., and Brunner, D.: Coronary atherosclerosis in cases of traumatic death. In *Physical Activity and Aging*. Vol. 4 of *Medicine and Sport*, ed. by D. Brunner and E. Jokl. White Plains, N.Y.: A.J. Phiebig, 1969, p. 241.

Moerl, H.: The increasing frequency of severe atherosclerosis. Zentralbl. Allg. Pathol., *115*:579–587, 1972. (Eng. Summary.)

Monteiro, L.A.: After heart attack: behavioral expectations for the cardiac. Soc. Sci. Med., 7:55, 1973.

Morris, J.N., and Crawford, M.D.: Coronary heart disease and physical activity of work. Br. Med. J., 2:1485, 1958.

Morris, J., et al.: Incidence and prediction of ischemic heart disease in London busmen. Lancet, 2:553, 1966.

Morris, J., et al.: CHD and physical activity of work. Lancet, 2:1111–1120, 1953.

Moss, A.J., et al.: Delay in hospitalization during the acute coronary period. Am. J. Cardiol., 24:659, 1969.

Neufeld, H.N.: Precursors of coronary arteriosclerosis in the pediatric and young adult age groups. Mod. Concepts Cardiovasc. Dis., 43:93–97, 1974.

Neufeld, H.N., et al.: Selected findings of Israeli ischemic heart disease study. Geriatrics, 28:134–136, 1973.

Paffenbarger, R.S., et al.: Work activity of longshoremen as related to death from CHD and stroke. N. Engl. J. Med., 282:1109–1114, 1970.

Parkinson, J., and Bedford, D.E.: Cardiac infarction and coronary thrombosis. Lancet, 4:4, 1928.

Paterson, J.C.: Stress, intimal hemorrhage and coronary occlusion. J. Occup. Med., 3:59–63, 1961.

Pell, S., and D'Alonzo, C.A.: A three-year study of myocardial infarction in a large employed population. JAMA, 175:463, 1961.

Pell, S., and D'Alonzo, C.A.: Immediate mortality and five year survival of employed men with a first myocardial infarction. N. Engl. J. Med., 270:915, 1964.

Quain, R.: On fatty diseases of the heart. (M. Chir. Tr., 33:121, 1850). In A Bibliography of Internal Medicine, Selected Diseases, ed. by A.L. Bloomfield. Chicago: University of Chicago Press, 1960, pp. 20–21.

Rechnitzer, P.A., et al.: Long term follow up study of survival and recurrence rates following myocardial infarction in exercising and control subject. Circulation, 45:853–857, 1972.

Richardson, P.J., Livesley, B., and Oram, S.: Angina pectoris with normal coronary arteries: transvenous myocardial biopsy in diagnosis. Lancet, 2:677–680, 1974.

Rose, G., Prineas, R.J., and Mitchell, J.R.: Myocardial infarction and the intrinsic calibre of coronary arteries. Br. Heart J., 29:548, 1967.

Shanoff, H.M., and Little, J.A.: Studies of male survivors of myocardial infarction due to essential atherosclerosis. I. Characteristics of the patients. Can. Med. Assoc. J., 84:519, 1961.

Shekelle, R.B., Ostfeld, A.M., and Paul, O.: Social status and incidence of coronary heart disease. J. Chronic Dis., 22:381, 1969.

Simon, A.B., et al.: Components of delay in the pre-hospital setting of acute myocardial infarction. Am. J. Cardiol., 30:475, 1972.

Spain, D.M., and Brades, V.A.: Sudden death from CHD, survival time, frequency of thrombi and cigarette smoking. Chest, 58:107–110, 1970.

Stamler, J.: Acute myocardial infarction—progress in primary prevention. Br. Heart J., 33(Suppl):145–153, 1971.

Stamler, J., et al.: Prevalence and incidence of coronary heart disease in strata of the labor force of a Chicago industrial corporation. J. Chronic Dis., 11:405, 1960.

Stamler, J., Kjelsberg, M., and Hall, Y.: Epidemiologic studies on cardiovascular-renal diseases: 1. analysis of mortality by age-race-sex-occupation. J. Chronic Dis., *12*:440, 1960.

Syme, S.L., Borhani, N.O., and Buechley, R.W.: Cultural mobility and coronary heart disease in an urban area. Am. J. Epidemiol., *82*:334, 1965.

Taylor, H.L.: Coronary heart disease in physically active and sedentary populations. J. Sports Med. Phys. Fitness, *2*:73–82, 1962.

Taylor, H.L., et al.: Coronary heart disease in selected occupations of American railroads in relation to physical activity. Circulation, *3*:202, 1959.

Thompson, P.L., et al.: Exercise during acute myocardial infarction: an experimental study. Cardiovasc. Res., *7*:642–648, 1973.

Thompson, T.: *Hearts.* Greenwich, Conn.: Fawcett Publications, Inc., 1971.

Thompson, A.J., and Froelicher, V.F.: Kugel's artery as a major collateral channel in severe coronary disease. Aerosp. Med., *45*:1276, 1974.

Titus, J.L.: What's in a plaque and why does it form. In *Coronary Heart Disease,* ed. by R. Gorlin. Morris Plains, N.J.: Warner-Chilcott Laboratories, 1972. pp. 26–27.

Veterans Administration Cooperative Study Group on Anti-Hypertensive Agents. Effects of treatment on morbidity in hypertension. JAMA, *213*:1143, 1970.

Wardwell, W.I.: A study of stress and coronary heart disease in an urban population. Bull. N.Y. Acad. Med., *49*:521–531, 1973.

Warshaw, L.J.: Chronic disease and employability: the physician's role. J. Am. Med. Wom. Assoc., *20*:1120, 1965.

Weiss, H.S., et al.; Physical activity and atherosclerosis in the adult chicken. J. Atheroscler. Res., *6*:407, 1966.

Wenger, N.: The early ambulation of patients after myocardial infarction. Cardiology, *58*:1, 1973.

Wenger, N.K., et al.: Uncomplicated myocardial infarction. JAMA, *224*:511, 1973.

Zohman, L.R., and Tobis, J.R.: *Cardiac Rehabilitation.* New York: Grune and Stratton, 1970.

Zukel, W.J., et al.: A short term community study of the epidemiology of coronary heart disease: a preliminary report on the North Dakota study. Am. J. Public Health, *49*:1630–1639, 1959.

HYPER- AND HYPOTHYROIDISM

Tersung, R.L., and Winded, W.: Exercise and thyroid function. Med. Sci. Sports, *7(1)*:20–26, 1975.

LABORATORY PROCEDURES

Calculation of Metabolic Cost: Supplement to Guidelines for Graded Exercise Testing and Exercise Prescription (on request), American College of Sports Medicine, 1440 Monroe Street, 3002 Stadium, Madison, Wisconsin 53706.

Consolazio, C., Johnson, R., and Pecora, L.: *Physiological Measurements of Metabolic Functions in Man.* New York: McGraw-Hill Company, 1963.

Karatun, O.: Exercise technician. In *Adult Fitness Cardiac Rehabilitation,* ed. by P.K. Wilson, Baltimore: University Park Press, 1975. pp. 295–309.

Marston, M.: Compliance with medical regimens: a review of the literature. Nurs. Res., *19*:312, 1970.

Methodologies for Metabolic Measurements. (A. Norton) CP-2 Beckman Instruments, Inc. Fullerton, California.

Sterilization of Pulmonary Function Equipment. Warren E. Collins, Inc., 220 Wood Road, Braintree, Massachusetts 02184.

Preparing the Patient for Stress Testing. Marquette Electronics, Inc., P.O. Box 8039, 8200 West Tower Avenue, Milwaukee, Wisconsin, 53223.

LEARNING AND DATA SYSTEMS

Au-Vid Learning System: *Cardiovascular Medical Terminology, Cardiovascular Disorders & Surgery.* Garden Grove, California: Au-Vid Incorporated, 1972.

Coronary Artery Disease: A New Medcom Total Learning System. Morris Plains, N.J.: Warner-Chilcott Laboratory, 1972.

Fox, S. (ed.): *Coronary Heart Disease.* Denver: International Medical Corp., 1970.

NUTRITION

Asher, W.L.: *Treating the Obese.* New York: Medcom Press, 1974.

Brown, J., et al.: Nutritional and epidemiologic factors related to heart disease. World Rev. Nutr. Diet., *12*:1–42, 1970.

Castelli, W.P., and Moran, R.F.: Lipid studies for assessing the risk of cardiovascular disease and hyperlipidemia. Hum. Pathol., *2(1)*:153–164, 1971.

Conner, W., and Connor, S.: The key role of nutrition factors in prevention of coronary heart disease. Prev. Med., *1(1)*:49–83, 1972.

Dietary Management of Hyperlipoproteinemia: A Handbook for Physicians. Bethesda: National Heart and Lung Institute, 1970.

Durnin, J.V.G.A.: The influence of nutrition on physical activity and cardiovascular health. Can. Med. Assoc. J., *96*:715–720, 1967.

Eshleman, R., and Soderquist, K. (eds.): *The American Heart Association Cookbook.* New York: David McKay Co., 1973.

Froelicher, V.F.: The dietary prevention of atherosclerosis. Am. Fam. Phys., *7*:79–85, 1973.

Konishi, F.: *Exercise Equivalents of Foods.* Carbondale, Ill.: Southern Illinois University Press, 1973.

LaRosa, J.: Hyperlipoproteinemia: diagnosis and clinical significance; dietary management and drug therapy. Postgrad. Med., *51(7)*:62–79, 1972; *52(1–2)*:128–131, 1972.

Miettinen, M., et al.: Effect of cholesterol-lowering diet on mortality from coronary heart disease and other causes. Lancet, *2*:835–838, 1972.

National Health Foundation of Australia: Dietary fat and coronary heart disease: a review. Med. J. Aust., *1*:1155–1160, 1971.

Robinson, C.H.: *Basic Nutrition and Diet Therapy.* ed. 3. New York: Macmillan, 1975.

Sharkey, B.: *Physiological Fitness and Weight Control.* Missoula, Montana: Mountain Press Publishing Company, 1974.

Stamler, J., and Epstein, F.: Coronary heart disease: risk factors as guides to preventive action. Prev. Med., *1(1)*:27–48, 1972.

Stevenson, J.A.F.: Exercise, food intake and health in experimental animals. Can. Med. Assoc. J., *96*:862, 1967.

Turpinen, O., et al.: Dietary prevention of coronary heart disease: long-term experiment. Am. J. Clin. Nutr., *21*:255, 1968.

PATHOPHYSIOLOGY; DRUG THERAPY

Aldinger, E.E., and Sohal, S.S.: Effects of digitoxin on the ultrastructural myocardial changes in the rat subjected to chronic exercise. Am. J. Cardiol., *26*:369–374, 1970.

Aldinger, E.E.: Effects of digitoxin on the development of cardiac hypertrophy in the rat subjected to chronic exercise. Am. J. Cardiol., *25*:339, 1970.

Bailey, I.K., et al.: Effect of beta-adrenergic blockade with propranolol on ST-segment suppression and circulatory dynamics during exercise in patients with effort angina. Am. Heart J., *92(4)*:416–426, 1976.

Berne, R., and Levy, M.: *Cardiovascular Physiology.* St. Louis: C. V. Mosby Company, 1967.

Bodenheimer, M.M., Banka, V.S., and Helfant, R.H.: Propranolol in experimental myocardial ischemia: dissociation of effects on contraction and epicardial ST segments. Am. Heart J., *92(4)*:481–486, 1976.

Briller, A.S., and Conn, L.H., Jr.: *The Myocardial Cell, Structure and Function and Modification by Drugs.* Philadelphia: University of Pennsylvania Press, 1966.

Brobeck, J.R.: *Best and Taylor's Physiological Basis of Medical Practice.* ed. 9. Baltimore: Williams and Wilkins Company, 1973.

Bruce, R.A.: The effects of digoxin on fatiguing static and dynamic exercise in man. Clin. Sci., *34*:29–33, 1968.

Detry, J., and Bruce, R.: Effects of nitroglycerine on "maximal" oxygen intake and exercise electrocardiogram in coronary heart disease. Circulation, *44*:390, 1971.

Frishman, W.H., et al.: Aspirin therapy in angina pectoris; effects on platelet aggregation, exercise tolerance and electrocardiographic manifestations of ischemia. Am. Heart J., *92(1)*:3–10, 1976.

Fowler, N.O., and Brest, A.: *Diagnostic Methods in Cardiology.* Philadelphia: F.A. Davis Company, 1975.

Guyton, A.: *Textbook of Medical Physiology.* Philadelphia: W. B. Saunders Company, 1971.

Hackett, T.P., et al.: Reduction of anxiety in the coronary care unit: a controlled double-blind comparison of chlordiazepoxide and amobarbital. Curr. Ther. Res., *14*:649, 1972.

Henning, H.: Beneficial effects of nitroglycerin on abnormal ventricular wall motion at rest and during exercise in patients with previous myocardial infarction. Am. J. Cardiol., *37*:623–629, 1976.

Hurst, J., et al.: *The Heart: Arteries and Veins.* ed. 3. New York: McGraw-Hill Book Company, Inc., 1974.

Kattus, A.A.: Physical training and heteradrenergic blocking drugs in modifying coronary insufficiency. In *Coronary Circulation and Energetics of the Myocardium,* ed. by G. Marchetti and B. Toccardi. New York: S. Karger AG, 1967.

Moir, D.C., et al.: Cardiotoxicity of amitriptyline. Lancet, *2:*561, 1972.

Moir, D.C.: Tricyclic antidepressants and cardiac disease. Am. Heart J., *86:*841, 1973.

McMahon, F.G., et al.: *Cardiovascular Drugs.* Mount Kisco, N.Y.: Futura Publishing Company, 1974.

Mountcastle, V.B., et al.: *Medical Physiology.* ed. 13. St. Louis: C. V. Mosby Co., 1974.

Parker, J.O., et al.: Effect of nitroglycerine ointment on the clinical and hemodynamic response to exercise. Am. J. Cardiol., *38:*162–166, 1976.

Physician's Desk Reference to Pharmaceutical Specialities and Biologicals. Published by Medical Economics Inc., Litton Publications Inc., Oradell, New Jersey. Annual Publication.

Robb, G.P., and Marks, H.H.: Latent coronary artery disease: determination of its presence and severity by the exercise electrocardiogram. Am. J. Cardiol., *13:*603, 1964.

Rushmer, R.F.: *Cardiovascular Dynamics.* ed. 4. Philadelphia: W. B. Saunders, 1976.

Wolf, G.L., et al.: *Practical Management of Hypertension.* Mount Kisco, N.Y.: Futura Publishing Company, 1975.

PHYSICAL FITNESS

Adams, C.W.: Introduction in symposium on exercise and the heart. Am. J. Cardiol., *30(7):*713–715, 1972.

Balke, B., and Ware, R.W.: An experimental study of physical fitness of Air Force personnel. U.S. Armed Forces Med. J., *10:*675–688, 1959.

Banister, E.W., Tomanek, R.J., and Cvorkov, N.: Ultrastructural modifications in rat heart: responses to exercise and training. Am. J. Physiol., *220:*1935, 1971.

Belloc, N., Breslow, L., and Hochstim, J.R.: Measurement of physical health in a general population survey. Am. J. Epidemiol., *93(5):*328, 1971.

Berger, R.A.: *Conditioning for Men.* Boston: Allyn & Bacon, Inc., 1973.

Cooper, K.H.: *The New Aerobics,* New York: M. Evans and Co., 1970.

Corbin, C., et al.: *Concepts in Physical Education.* Dubuque: Wm. C. Brown Publishers, 1975.

Fox, E.L., and Mathews, D.K.: *Interval Training: Conditioning for Sports and General Fitness.* Philadelphia: W. B. Saunders Co., 1974.

Hockey, R.V.: *Physical Fitness: the Pathway to Healthful Living.* St. Louis: C. V. Mosby Co., 1973.

Kusinitz, I., et al.: *The Challenge of Physical Fitness.* Westport, Conn.: Physical Fitness Laboratory, Ltd, 1969.

Lurie, J.Z., and Segev, S.: *The Israel Army Physical Fitness Book.* New York: Grosset and Dunlap. 1969.

Myers, C.R.: *The Official YMCA Physical Fitness Handbook.* New York: Popular Library, 1975.

Myers, C.R.L., Golding, A., and Sinning, W.E.: *The Y's Way to Physical Fitness.* Emmaus, Pa.: Rodale Press, 1973.

Opie, L.: Sudden death and sport. Lancet, *1*:263, 1975.

Paul, O.: Physical activity and coronary heart disease. Am. J. Cardiol., *23*:303–306, 1969.

Shephard, R.J.: Sudden death—a significant hazard of exercise. Br. J. Med., *8*:101, 1974.

Spackman, R.R.: *Exercise in the Office.* Carbondale, Ill.: Southern Illinois University Press, 1968.

Swengros, G.: *Fitness with Glenn Swengros.* New York: Hawthorne Books, Inc., 1971.

Taylor, H.L., et al.: Death rates among physically active and sedentary employees of the railroad industry. Am. J. Public Health, *52*:1697, 1962.

Vitale, F.: *Individualized Fitness Programs.* New Jersey: Prentice-Hall, Inc., 1973.

Weinberger, C.W.: Remarks, National Conference of Physical Fitness in Business and Industry. Washington, D.C., 1973. pp. 3–4

RISK FACTORS

Barboriak, J.J., et al: Risk factors in patients undergoing aorta-coronary bypass surgery. J. Thorac. Cardiovasc. Surg., *64*:92–97, 1972.

Barcenas, C., Hoeffler, H.P., and Lie, J.T.: Obesity, football, dog days and siriasis: a deadly combination. Am. Heart J.: *92(2)*:237–244, 1976.

Berkson, D.M., et al.: Heart rate: an important risk factor for coronary mortality, ten year experience of the People's Gas Co. In *Atherosclerosis; Proceedings Second International Symposium.* ed. by R.J. Jones. New York: Springer-Verlag, 1970. pp. 382–389.

Chapman, J.M., and Massey, F.J.: The interrelationship of serum cholesterol, hypertension, body weight and risk of coronary disease. J. Chronic Dis., *17*:933, 1964.

Chiang, B.N., Perlman, L.V., and Epstein, F.H.: Overweight and hypertension. Circulation, *39*:403, 1969.

Cooper, K.H., et al.: Physical fitness levels vs. selected coronary risk factors. JAMA, *236*:166–169, 1976.

Dick, T.B.S., and Stone, M.C.: Prevalence of three cardiac risk factors in a random sample of men and in patients with ischemic heart disease. Br. Heart J., *35*:381–385, 1973.

Deutscher, S., Epstein, F.H., and Keller, J.B.: Relationship between familial aggregation of CHD and risk factors in the general population. Am. J. Epidemiol., *69*:510–520, 1969.

Friedman, M., and Rosenman, R.H.: Type A behavior pattern, its association with CHD. Ann. Clin. Res., *3*:300–312, 1971.

Froelicher, V.F., and Oberman, A.: Analysis of epidemiologic studies of physical inactivity as risk factor for coronary artery disease. Prog. Cardiovasc. Dis., *14*:41, 1972.

Garbus, S.B., and Reynolds, J.L.: The first mass hypertensive screening in a major city. (Abstract). Circulation, *48(Suppl. IV)*:IV–93, 1973.

Goldrick, R.B.,Sinnett, P.F., and Whyte, H.M.: An assessment of coronary heart disease and coronary risk factors in a New Guinea highland population. In *Atherosclerosis, Proceedings Second International Symposium,* ed. by R.J. Jones, New York: Springer-Verlag, 1970. pp. 366–373.

Hammond, E.C.: Smoking in relation to the death rates of one million men and women. In *Epidemiological Approaches to the Study of Cancer and Other Diseases.* Nat. Cancer Institute Monograph No. 19. Bethesda: U.S. Public Health Service, 1966, pp. 127–204.

Heyden, S., et al.: Body weight and cigarette smoking as risk factors. Arch. Intern. Med., *128*:916–919, 1971.

Intersociety Commission for Heart Diseases: Hypertension study group report. Circulation, *42*:A-39–41, 1970.

Kahn, H.A.: The incidence of hypertension and associated factors, Israel ischemic heart disease study. Am. Heart J., *84*:171–182, 1972.

Kannel, W.B., et al.: Relation of body weight to development of coronary heart disease. Circulation, *35*:734–744, 1967.

Kannel, W.B., Gordon, T., and Schwartz, M.J.: Systolic versus diastolic blood pressure and risk of coronary heart disease. Am. J. Cardiol., *27*:335–346, 1971.

Kannel, W.B., et al.: Risk factors in coronary heart disease, an evaluation of several serum lipids as predictors of coronary heart disease, the Framingham study. Ann. Intern. Med., *61*:888–898, 1964.

Kennedy, R.F.: Setting the theme. In *Proceedings, 1967 World Conference on Smoking and Health.* ed. by H.A. Goodman. New York: American Cancer Society, 1967. pp. 4–13.

Khosla, T., and Lowe, C.R.: Indices of obesity from body weight and height. Br. J. Prev. Med., *21*:122–128, 1967.

Montoye, H.J., et al.: Fitness, fatness and serum cholesterol; an epidemiological study of an entire community. Res. Qtr., *47(3)*:400–408, 1976.

Myasnikov, A.L.: Influence of some factors on development of experimental cholesterol atherosclerosis. Circulation, *17*:99, 1958.

National Center for Health Statistics: Cigarette smoking and health characteristics. Washington, D.C.: US Health Service Publication, No. 1000, Series 10, No. 34, 1967. pp. 12–14.

Naughton, J., and Bruhn, J.: Emotional stress, physical activity and ischemic heart disease. DM, July:1, 1970.

Pesonen, E., Norio, R., and Sarna, S.: Thickenings in the coronary arteries in infancy as an indication of genetic factors in coronary heart disease. Circulation, *51*:218, 1975.

Rose, G.A., and Blackburn, H.: Cardiovascular survey methods. Geneva: World Health Organization, 1968.

Rosenman, R.H., et al.: A study of comparative blood pressure measures in predicting risk of coronary heart disease. Circulation, *54*:51–58, 1976.

Seltzer, C.C.: Overweight and obesity, the associated cardiovascular risk. Minn. Med. J., *52*:1265–1270, 1969.

Stamler, J.: The scientific background. In *Proceedings, 1967 World Conference on Smoking and Health.* ed. by H.A. Goodman. New York: American Cancer Society, 1967. pp. 44–73.

Taylor, C.B., et al.: Risk factors in the pathogenesis of atherosclerotic heart disease and generalized atherosclerosis. Ann. Clin. Lab. Sci., *2*:239, 1972.

Tyroler, H.A., et al.: Blood pressure and cholesterol as CHD risk factors. Arch. Intern. Med., *128*:907–914, 1971.

THERAPEUTIC EXERCISE

Acker, J.E.: Exercise programs aiding in primary prevention or rehabilitation of heart disease. Malattie Card., *10*:457–459, 1969.

Ad Hoc Committee on Habilitation of the Young Cardiac, American Heart Assoc.: Activity guidelines for young patients with heart disease. Phys. Sports Med., *8*:47, 1876.

Blazek, W.V., and Player, J.: A telemetry study of nine cardiac patients while swimming and running. Unpublished manuscript. University of Illinois, Abraham Lincoln School of Medicine, 1971.

Blazina, M.: Orthopedic problems seen in exercise programs. Nebr. State Med. J., *57*:477–479, 1972.

Blocker, W.P.: Physical activities—teaming up patients and programs. Postgrad. Med., *60*:56, 1976.

Bonanno, J.A., Lies, J.E., and Mason, D.T.: Effects of exercise training on coronary risk factors. Circulation, *48(Suppl. IV)*:IV–93, 1973.

Boyer, J., and Kasch, F.: Exercise therapy in hypertensive men. JAMA, *211*:1668–1671, 1970.

Boyer, J., and Kasch, F.: Changes in maximum work capacity resulting from six months training in patients with ischemic heart disease. Med. Sci. Sports, *1*:156–159, 1969.

Boyer, J.L.: Physical activity programs following myocardial infarction. Hosp. Med., *8*:95–111, 1972.

Brock, L.: Early reconditioning for post myocardial patients: Spalding Rehabilitation Center. In *Exercise Testing and Exercise Training in Coronary Heart Disease.* ed. by. J. Naughton and H.K.Hellerstein. New York: Academic Press, 1973. pp. 315–335.

Brock, L.L.: Rehabilitation of the myocardial infarction patient. In *Coronary Heart Disease, Prevention, Detection, Rehabilitation with Emphasis on Exercise Testing.* ed. by. S.M. Fox. Denver: International Medical Corp., 1974. pp. 601–610.

Bruce, E.H., et al.: Comparison of active participants and dropouts in CAPRI cardiopulmonary rehabilitation programs. Am. J. Cardiol., *37*:22, 1976.

Bruce, R.A.: The benefits of physical training for patients with coronary heart disease. In *Controversy in Internal Medicine II*, ed. by F.J. Ingelfinger, et al. Philadelphia: W.B. Saunders, 1974.

Bruce, R.A., et al.: Separation of effects of cv disease and age on ventricular function with exercise. Am. J. Cardiol., *34*:757–762, 1974.

Bruce, R.A., Hornstein, T., and Blackman, J.: Myocardial infarction after normal response to exercise. Circulation, *38*:552–555, 1968.

Brunner, D., and Maneus, G.: Physical activity at work and ischemic heart disease. In *Coronary Heart Disease and Physical Fitness,* by. O.A. Larsen and R.O. Malmborg. Baltimore: University Park Press, 1971. pp. 244–268.

Brunner, D.: The influence of physical activity on incidence and prognosis of ischemic heart disease. *Prevention of Ischemic Heart Disease,* ed. W. Raab. Springfield, Ill.: Charles C Thomas, 1966.

Buck, R.L.: It's only a sprained ankle. Am. Fam. Physician, *6(4)*:69–75, October, 1975.

Cain, H.D., Frasher, W.G., and Stivelman, R.: Graded activity program for safe return to self-care after myocardial infarction. JAMA, *177*:111–115, 1961.

Cantwell, J.D., and Fletcher, G.F.: Cardiac complications while jogging. JAMA, *210*:130, 1969.

Cantwell, J.D., et al.: Dynamic exercise training in post myocardial infarction patients. Med. Sci. Sports, *5*:66–67, 1973.

Clausen, J., and Trap-Jensen, J.: Effects of training on the distribution of cardiac output in patients with coronary artery disease. Circulation, *42*:611, 1970.

Clausen, J., and Trap-Jensen, J.: Heart rate and arterial blood pressure during exercise in patients with angina pectoris. Circulation, *53*:436–442, 1976.

Cobb, F.R., Ruby, R.L., and Fariss, B.L.: Effects of exercise on acute coronary occlusion in dogs with prior partial occlusion. (Abstract) Circulation, *37 and 38*:104, 1968.

Collins, R.: Reconstruction of the athlete's injured knee: anatomy, diagnosis, treatment. Orthop. Clin. North Am., *2(1)*:207–208, March, 1971.

Conner, J.F., et al.: Effects of exercise on coronary collateralization—angiographic studies of six patients in a supervised exercise program. Med. Sci. Sports, *8(3)*:145–151, 1976.

Cooper, D.L., and Fair, J.: Rehabilitation through underwater exercise. Phys. Sports Med., *4*:143, 1976.

Costill, D.L., et al.: Physical training in men with coronary heart disease. Med. Sci. Sports, *6*:70, 1974.

Crabbe, W.: *Orthopedics for the Undergraduate.* Philadelphia: Lea & Febiger, 1969.

Croog, S.H., et al.: The heart patient and the recovery process. Soc. Sci. Med., *2*:111, 1968.

Cyriax, J.: *Textbook of Orthopedic Medicine Vol. 1, Diagnosis of Soft Tissue Lesions.* Baltimore: Williams & Wilkins Company, 1969.

Detry, J.M.R., et al.: Increased arteriovenous oxygen difference after physical training in coronary heart disease. Circulation, *44*:44–109, 1971.

Douglas, J.E.: Cardiovascular conditioning and rehabilitation, a mandate for action. J. Arkansas Med. Soc., *69*:173–177, 1974.

Fisher, S.: Impact of physical disability on vocational activity: work status following myocardial infarction. Scand. J. Rehabil. Med., *2*:65, 1970.

Fletcher, G.F., and Cantwell, J.D.: Outpatient gym exercise program for patients with recent myocardial infarction. Arch. Intern. Med., *134*:63, 1974.

Fletcher, G.F., and Cantwell, J.D.: *Exercise in the Management of Coronary Heart Disease.* Springfield, Ill.: Charles C Thomas, 1971.

Fox, S.M., Naughton, J.P., and Gorman, P.A.: Physical activity and cardiovascular health I. Potential for prevention of CHD and possible mechanism. Mod. Concepts Cardiovasc. Dis., *41*:17–20, 1972.

Fox, S.M., Naughton, J.P., and Gorman, P.A.: Physical activity and cardiovascular health, II. The exercise prescription: frequency and type of exercise. Mod. Concepts Cardiovasc. Dis., *41*:25–30, 1972.

Fox, S.M.: Physical activity and changing the risk of coronary heart disease. In *Coronary Heart Disease, Prevention, Detection, Rehabilitation with Emphasis on Exercise Testing,* ed. by S.M. Fox. Denver: International Medical Corp., 1974.

Fox, S.M., and Haskell, W.L.: Physical activity and health maintenance. J. Rehabil., *32*:89–92, 1966.

Fox, S.M., and Naughton, J.P.: Physical activity and prevention of CHD. Prev. Med., *1*:92–120, 1972.

Fox, S.M., Naughton, J.P., and Haskell, W.L.: Physical activity and the prevention of CHD. Ann. Clin. Res., *3*:404–432, 1971.

Frank, C.W., et al.: Physical inactivity as a lethal factor in myocardial infarction among men. Circulation, *34*:1022, 1966.

Frick, M. and Katila, M.: Hemodynamic consequences of physical training after myocardial infarction. Circulation, *37*:192, 1968.

Gertler, M.M.: Ischemic heart disease, heredity and body build as affected by exercise. In *Proceedings of the International Symposium on Physical Activity and Cardiovascular Health*. Toronto, Ontario, 1966. pp. 728–732.

Gottheiner, V.: Long range strenuous sports training for cardiac reconditioning and rehabilitation. Am. J. Cardiol., *22*:426–435, 1968.

Gyntelberg, F.: Physical fitness and coronary heart disease, male residents in Copenhagen, aged 40–59. Dan. Med. Bull., *20*:1–4, 1973.

Haskell, W.L.: Physical activity and the prevention of coronary heart disease: what type exercise might be effective. J. S.C. Med. Assoc., *65*:41–45, 1969.

Hay, D.R.: Rehabilitation after myocardial infarction and acute coronary insufficiency. N. Z. Med. J., *71*:267, 1970.

Heller, E.M.: Rehabilitation after myocardial infarction: practical experience with a graded exercise program. Can. Med. Assoc. J., *97*:22–27, 1967.

Hellerstein, H.K., and Hornstein, T.R.: Assessing and preparing the patient for return to a meaningful productive life. J. Rehabil., *32*:43–58, 1966.

Hellerstein, H.K.: Effects of an active physical reconditioning intervention program on the clinical course of coronary artery disease. Mal. Cardiovasc.. (Firenze), *10*:461, 1969.

Hellerstein, H.K., et al.: Discussion on heart disease and athletics. Phys. Sports Med., *4*:66–69, 1976.

Hellerstein, H.K., and Goldstone, E.: Rehabilitation of patients with heart disease. Postgrad. Med., *15*:265–279, 1954.

Hellerstein, H.K., and Ford, A.B.: Rehabilitation of the cardiac patient. JAMA, *164*:225, 1957.

Hellerstein, H.K., et al.: The effect of physical activity, a community program and study among patients and normal coronary prone subjects. Minn. Med., *52*:1341–1355, 1969.

Hellerstein, H., et al.: The influence of active conditioning upon subjects with coronary heart disease. Can. Med. Assoc. J., *96*:758, 1967.

Hinkle, L.E., et al.: Occupation, education and coronary heart disease. Science, *161*:238–245, 1968.

Hirsch, E.Z., Hellerstein, H.K., and MacLeod, C.A.: Physical training and coronary disease. In *Exercise and the Heart, Guidelines for Exercise Programs*, ed. by R.L. Morse. Springfield, Ill.: Charles C Thomas Publisher, 1972. pp. 106–187.

Hyman, M.D.: Social isolation and performance in rehabilitation. J. Chronic Dis., *25*:85, 1972.

Jokl, E., and McClellan, J.T.: Exercise and cardiac death. In *Medicine and Sport*, Vol. V. Baltimore: University Park Press, 1971.

Kannel, W.B.: Physical exercise and lethal ASD. N. Engl. J. Med., *282*:1153, 1970.

Kannel, W.B., Sorlie, P., and McNamara, P.: The relation of physical activity to risk of coronary heart disease: the Framingham study. In *Coronary Heart Disease and Physical Fitness,* ed. by O.A. Larsen and R.O. Malmborg. Baltimore: University Park Press, 1971, p. 256.

Kaplinsky, E., et al.: Effects of physical training in dogs with coronary artery ligation. Circulation, *37*:556, 1968.

Katz, L.N.: Physical fitness and CHD—some basic views. Circulation, *35*:405–414, 1967.

Kavanagh, T., Shephard, R.H., and Pandit, V.: Marathon running after myocardial infarction. JAMA, *229*:1602, 1974.

Kellermann, J.J., et al.: Return to work after myocardial infarction, comparative study of rehabilitated and non-rehabilitated patients. Geriatrics, *23*:151–156, 1968.

Kellermann, J.J.: Physical conditioning in patients after myocardial infarction. Schweiz Med. Wschr., *103*:79–85, 1973.

Keys, A.: Physical activity and the epidemiology of coronary heart disease. Med. Sports, *4*:250–266, 1970.

Keys, A., et al.: Coronary heart disease among Minnesota business and professional men followed 15 years. Circulation, *28*:381–395, 1963.

Klafs, C., and Arnheim, D.: *Modern Principles of Athletic Training: The Science of Injury, Prevention and Care.* St. Louis: C. V. Mosby Company, 1973.

Kouchoukos, N.T., and Karp, R.B.: Management of the postoperative cardiovascular surgical patient. Am. Heart J., *92(4)*:513–531, 1976.

Krause, E.: Structured strain in a marginal profession: rehabilitation counseling. J. Health Hum. Behav., *6*:55, 1965.

Krehl, W.A.: The basis for a preventive cardiovascular program. J. Occup. Med., *15*:45–47, 1973.

Larsen, A.O., and Malmborg, R.O.: *Coronary Heart Disease and Physical Fitness.* Baltimore: University Park Press, 1971.

Leon, A.S.: Comparative cardiovascular adaptation to exercise in animals and man and its relevance to coronary heart disease. In *Comparative Pathophysiology of Circulatory Disturbances,* ed. by C. Bloor. New York: Plenum Publishing Corp. 1974. p. 143.

Licht, S., and Johnson, E.: *Therapeutic Exercise.* Baltimore: Waverly Press Inc., 1965.

McAllister, F.F., Bertsch, R., and Jacobson, J.: The accelerating effect of muscular exercise on experimental atherosclerosis. Arch. Surg., *80*:54, 1959.

McPherson, B.D., et al.: Psychological effects of an exercise program for post-infarct and normal adult men. J. Sport Med., *7*:95–102, 1967.

Morris, J.N., et al.: Vigorous exercise in leisure time and the incidence of CHD. Lancet, *1*:333–339, 1973.

Morris, J.N., et al.; Coronary heart disease and physical activity of work. Lancet, *2*:1053–1057, 1953.

Morris, J.N.: Occupation and coronary heart disease. Arch. Intern. Med., *194*:903–907, 1959.

Mulcahy, R., et al.: The rehabilitation of patients with coronary heart disease. Scand. J. Rehabil. Med., *2*:108, 1970.

Naughton, J., Bruhn, J., and Lategola, M.T.: Rehabilitation following myocardial infarction. Am. J. Med., *46*:725–734, 1969.

Naughton, J.P., and McCoy, J.F.: Observations on the relationship of physical activity to the serum cholesterol concentration of healthy men and cardiac patients. J. Chronic Dis., *19*:727, 1966.

Pederson, B.O.: The effect of physical training in myocardial infarction. In *Coronary Heart Disease and Physical Fitness*, ed. by R.O. Malmborg and O.A. Larsen. Baltimore: University Park Press, 1971. pp. 115–116.

Pyfer, H., et al.: Group exercise rehabilitation for cardiopulmonary patients, a five year study. Med. Sci. Sports, *5*:71, 1973.

Pyorala, K. et al.: A controlled study on the effects of 18 months physical training in sedentary middle-aged men with indices of risk relative to coronary heart disease. In *Coronary Heart Disease and Physical Fitness*, ed. by O.A. Larsen and R.O. Malmborg. Baltimore: University Park Press, 1971, p. 261.

Rechnitzer, P.A., et al.: Effects of 24 week exercise program on normal adults and patients with previous myocardial infarction. Br. Med. J., *1*:734–735, 1967.

Redwood, D.R., Rosing, D.R., and Epstein, S.E.: Circulatory and symptomatic effects of physical training in patients with coronary artery disease and angina pectoris. N. Engl. J. Med., *286*:959–965, 1972.

Richard, A.P.: Effect of training on myocardial mitochondria. Med. Sci. Sports, *4*:64, 1972.

Rousseau, M.F., Brasseur, L.A., and Detry, J.M.R.: Hemodynamic determinants of maximal oxygen intake in patients with healed myocardial infarction: influence of physical training. Circulation, *43*:943–949, 1973.

Rudd, J.J., and Day, W.C.: A physical fitness program for patients with hypertension. J. Am. Geriatr. Soc., *15*:373, 1967.

Rumbaugh, D.M.: Rehabilitation psychological aspects. J. Rehabil. *32*:56–58, 1966.

Safillos-Rothschild, C.: The self-definitions of the disabled and implications for rehabilitation. G. Albrecht ed. *Socialization in Disability Process*. ed. by G. Albrecht. Pittsburgh: University of Pittsburgh Press, 1974.

Sanne, H.M., and Wilhelmsen, L.: Physical activity as prevention and therapy in CHD. Scand. J. Rehabil. Med., *3*:47–56, 1971.

Sanne, H., Elmfeldt, D., and Wilhelmsen, L.: Preventive effect of physical training after a myocardial infarction. In *Preventive Cardiology*, ed. by G. Tibblin et al. New York: John Wiley & Sons, 1972.

Sanne, H.: Exercise tolerance and physical training of non-selected patients after myocardial infarction. Acta Med. Scand. Suppl., *551*:1–124, 1973.

Scheuer, J.: Physical training and intrinsic cardiac adaptation. Circulation, *47*:677–680, 1973.

Shkhvatsabaya, I.K., and Zaitsev, V.P.: Psychological factors in myocardial infarction and problems of rehabilitation. Ter. Arkh., *44*:22–27, 1972. (Eng. Summary)

Simonson, E.: Evaluation of cardiac performance in exercise. Am. J. Cardiol., *30*:722–726, 1972.

Spain, D.M., and Bradess, V.A.: Occupational physical activity and the degree of coronary atherosclerosis in "normal" men. Circulation, *22*:239, 1960.

Stone, W.J.: The effects of physical training on post-coronary patients. (Abstr) Research papers, AAHPER Convention, 1972, p. 63.

Taggart, P., Parkinson, P., and Carruthers, M.: Cardiac responses to thermal, physical and emotional stress. Br. Med. J., *3*:71–76, 1972.

Tepperman, J., and Pearlman, D.: Effects of exercise and anemia on coronary arteries of small animals as revealed by the Corrison-Cast technique. Circ. Res., 9:576–579, 1961.

Varnauskas, E., et al.: Haemodynamic effects of physical training on coronary patients. Lancet, 2:8–12, 1966.

Wenger, N.K.: Benefits of a rehabilitation program following myocardial infarction. Geriatrics, 28:64–67, 1973.

Wenger, N.K.: Coronary care—rehabilitation after myocardial infarction. Prepared for the Coronary Care Committee, Council on Clinical Cardiology and the Committee on Medical Education. American Heart Association, New York, November, 1973.

Werko, L.: Clinical value of physical conditioning in patients with manifest CHD. In *Coronary Heart Disease and Physical Fitness*, ed. by O.A. Larsen and R.O. Malmborg. Baltimore: University Park Press, 1971, pp 13–15.

Whitsett, T.L., and Naughton, J.: The effect of exercise on systolic time intervals in sedentary and active individuals and rehabilitated patients with heart disease. Am. J. Cardiol., 27:352–358, 1971.

Wilson, P. K.: Etiologic and initial cardiovascular characteristics of participants in a cardiac rehabilitation program. J. Am. Corr. Ther. Soc., 27(4):122, 1973.

Zohman, L.R.: Cardiac rehabilitation: its role in evaluation and management of the patient with coronary heart disease. Am. Heart J., 85(5):706–710, 1973.

Zohman, L.R., and Tobis, J.S.: The effect of exercise training on patients with angina pectoris. Arch. Phys. Med., 48:525–526, 1967.

appendix **B**

Sources of Patient Education Materials

American Heart Association
7320 Greenville Ave.
Dallas, Texas 75231

American Hospital Association
840 North Lake Shore Drive
Chicago, Illinois 60611

Au-Vid Corporated
P. O. Box 964
Garden Grove, California 92642

Concept Media
1500 Adams Avenue
Costa Mesa, California 92626

Ives Laboratory, Inc.
685 Third Avenue
New York, New York 10017

Medfact
420 Lake Avenue N. E.
Massillon, Ohio 44646

Merck Sharp & Dohme
Division of Merck and Co., Inc.
West Point, Pa.   19486

Metropolitan Life Insurance Co.
1 Madison Avenue
New York, New York   10010

Milner Fenwick, Inc.
3800 Liberty Heights Avenue
Baltimore, Maryland   21215

National High Blood Pressure Program
High Blood Pressure Information Center
120/80 National Institute of Health
Landow Building, Room 1012
Bethesda, Maryland   20014

Pritchett & Hull Associates
2996 Grandview Avenue N. E.
Atlanta, Georgia   30305

Prudential Insurance Co.
Public Relations & Advertising
Newark, New Jersey   07102

Public Inquiries & Reports Branch
National Heart & Lung Institute
Bethesda, Maryland   20014

Research Media, Inc.
4 Medland Avenue
Hicksville, New York   11801

Robert J. Brady Company
Bowie, Maryland   20715

Sharing and Caring Booklet
Southwestern Connecticut Heart Association
15 Bettswood Road
Newark, Connecticut   06851

Trainex Corporation Subsidiary Medcom, Inc.
P. O. Box 116
Garden Grove, California   92642

U. S. Department of H. E. W.
Health Resources Administration
Division of Facilities Utilization
Consultation on Hospital Functions Branch
5600 Fishers Lane
Rockville, Maryland   20852

Video Learning Systems
P. O. Box 1
Eau Claire, Wisconsin   54701

Wisconsin Heart Association
205 W. Highland Avenue
Milwaukee, Wisconsin   53203

appendix C

Involved Agencies

1. American Alliance for Health, Physical Education and Recreation, 1201 Sixteenth St. N.W., Washington, D.C.
2. American Association of Fitness Directors in Business and Industry, President's Council on Physical Fitness and Sports, Washington, D.C.   20201
3. American College of Cardiology, 9650 Rockville Pike, Bethesda, Md.   20014
4. American College of Sports Medicine, 1440 Monroe St., Madison, Wis.   53706
5. American Heart Association, 7320 Greenville Ave., Dallas, Texas   75231
6. American Medical Association, 535 No. Dearborn St., Chicago, Ill.   60610
7. Canadian Association for Health, Physical Education and Recreation, 333 River Road, Vanier City, Ontario, KIL 8B9, Canada
8. Canadian Heart Foundation, 1130 Bay Street, Toronto 5, Ontario, Canada
9. Canadian Medical Association, 129 Adelaide Street West, Toronto, Canada
10. Fitness & Amateur Sports Directorate, Department of Health and Welfare, Brooke Clayton Building, Ottawa, Canada
11. Fitness Finders, Inc., 22 Main Street, Emmaus, Pa.   18049
12. National Council of Y.M.C.A.s of Canada, 2160 Yonge Street, Toronto 295, Ontario, Canada
13. National Council of Y.M.C.A. of U.S.A., Director of Physical Fitness, 40 W. Long Street, Columbus, Ohio   43200
14. National Jogging Association, Suite 513, Washington Medical Bldg., Champaign, Ill.   61820
15. President's Council on Physical Fitness, Washington, D.C.   20202

Graded Exercise Test (GXT) Protocols

*Astrand Bicycle Test**

I. Preliminary Data   Subject_____
    Resting Heart Rate _____   Resting Blood Pressure____/____
    Age _____   Test Administrator(s)_____
II. Exercise Test**

Stage	RPM	Duration (minutes)	Workload (Kg) Female	Male	Heart Rate		Blood Pressure	
1	50	6	300 (1.9 met)	600 (2.38 met)	_____ 2nd min. _____ 4th min. _____ 6th min.		_____ / 2nd min. _____ / 4th min. _____ / 6th min.	
2	50	6	450 (2.14 met)	900 (2.86 met)	_____ 8th min. _____ 10th min. _____ 12th min.		_____ / 8th min. _____ / 10th min. _____ / 12th min.	
3	50	6	600 (2.38 met)	1200 (3.33 met)	_____ 14th min. _____ 16th min. _____ 18th min.		_____ / 14th min. _____ / 16th min. _____ / 18th min.	
Recovery			2 min. 4 min. 6 min. 8 min.		_____ _____ _____ _____		_____ / _____ / _____ / _____ /	

Comments:

*Adapted from Astrand, P. O., and I. Rhyming: Nomogram for calculation of aerobic capacity (physical fitness) from pulsenotes during sub-maximal work. J. Appl. Physiol., 7:218, 1954.
**End Point: Reaching a pre-set submaximal heart rate level.

Balke (Standard) Treadmill Test*

I. Preliminary Data   Subject_____
    Resting Heart Rate _____   Resting Blood Pressure ___/___
    Age _____   Test Administrator(s)_____
II. Graded Exercise Test

Stage	Duration (minutes)	Time (minutes)	Speed (mph & m/min)		Grade (%)	Mets	Heart Rate	Blood Pressure
1	2	1–2	3	80.5	2.5	4.32	_____	___/___
2	"	3–4	"	"	5.0	5.36	_____	___/___
3	"	5–6	"	"	7.5	6.39	_____	___/___
4	"	7–8	"	"	10.0	7.43	_____	___/___
5	"	9–10	"	"	12.5	8.46	_____	___/___
6	"	11–12	"	"	15.0	9.49	_____	___/___
7	"	13–14	"	"	17.5	10.53	_____	___/___
8	"	15–16	"	"	20.0	11.56	_____	___/___
9	"	17–18	"	"	22.5	12.59	_____	___/___
10	"	19–20	"	"	25.0	13.62	_____	___/___
11	"	21–22	"	"	27.5	14.65	_____	___/___
12	"	23–24	"	"	30.0	15.68	_____	___/___
Recovery		2 minutes			sitting		_____	___/___
		4 minutes			"		_____	___/___
		6 minutes			"		_____	___/___
		8 minutes			"		_____	___/___

Comments:

*Adapted from Balke, B., and R. W. Ware: An experimental study of physical fitness of Air Force personnel. U. S. Armed Forces Med. J., 10:675, 1959.

Balke (Substandard) Treadmill Test*

I. Preliminary Data   Subject_____
    Resting Heart Rate _____ Resting Blood Pressure ___/___
    Age _____   Test Administrator(s)_____
II. Graded Exercise Test

Stage	Duration (minutes)	Time (minutes)	Speed (mph & m/min)		Grade (%)	Mets	Heart Rate	Blood Pressure
1	2	1–2	2	53.6	0	2.53	_____	___/___
2	"	3–4	"	"	2.5	3.22	_____	___/___
3	"	5–6	"	"	5.0	3.91	_____	___/___
4	"	7–8	"	"	7.5	4.6	_____	___/___
5	"	9–10	"	"	10.0	5.29	_____	___/___
6	"	11–12	"	"	12.5	5.8	_____	___/___
7	"	13–14	"	"	15.0	6.67	_____	___/___
8	"	15–16	"	"	17.5	7.36	_____	___/___
9	"	17–18	"	"	20.0	8.04	_____	___/___
10	"	19–20	"	"	22.5	8.73	_____	___/___

Recovery	2 minutes		sitting	_____	_____
	4 minutes		"	_____	___/___
	6 minutes		"	_____	___/___
	8 minutes		"	_____	___/___

Comments:

*Personal communication.

Bruce Treadmill Test

I. Preliminary Data   Subject_____
    Resting Heart Rate _____ Resting Blood Pressure ___/___
    Age _____   Test Administrator(s)_____
II. Graded Exercise Test

Stage	Duration (minutes)	Time (minutes)	Speed (mph & m/min)		Grade (%)	Mets	Heart Rate	Blood Pressure
1	3	1–3	1.7	45.6	10	4.64	_____	___/___
2	"	4–6	2.5	67.0	12	7.05	_____	___/___
3	"	7–9	3.4	91.2	14	6.17	_____	___/___
4	"	10–12	4.2	112.6	16	13.48	_____	___/___
5	"	13–15	5.0	134.1	18	17.25	_____	___/___
6	"	16–18	5.5	147.5	20	20.39	_____	___/___
7	"	19–21	6.0	160.9	22	23.8	_____	___/___
Recovery		2 minutes			sitting		_____	
		4 minutes			"		_____	___/___
		6 minutes			"		_____	___/___
		8 minutes			"		_____	___/___

Comments:

*Bruce, R.A., Exercise Testing of Patients with Coronary Disease, Ann. Clin. Res., *3*:323, 1971.

Edgett (Diagnostic) Treadmill Test

I. Preliminary Data   Subject_____
    Resting Heart Rate _____   Resting Blood Pressure ____/____
    Age _____   Test Administrator(s)_____

II. Graded Exercise Test

Stage	Duration (minutes)	Time (minutes)	Speed (mph & m/min)		Grade (%)	Mets	Heart Rate	Blood Pressure
1	2	1–2	1.5	40.2	10	4.22	_____	____/____
2	"	3–4	2.0	53.6	12.5	5.98	_____	____/____
3	"	5–6	2.5	67.0	15	8.08	_____	____/____
4	"	7–8	3.0	80.5	15	9.5	_____	____/____
5	"	9–10	3.5	93.8	15	10.92	_____	____/____
6	"	11–12	4.0	107.3	15	12.34	_____	____/____
7	"	13–14	4.5	120.7	15	13.76	_____	____/____
Recovery		2 minutes			sitting		_____	_____
		4 minutes			"		_____	____/____
		6 minutes			"		_____	____/____
		8 minutes			"		_____	____/____

Comments:

Ellestad Treadmill Test*

I. Preliminary Data   Subject_____
    Resting Heart Rate _____ Resting Blood Pressure ___/___
    Age _____   Test Administrator(s)_____
II. Graded Exercise Test

Stage	Duration (minutes)	Time (minutes)	Speed (mph & m/min)		Grade (%)	Mets	Heart Rate	Blood Pressure
1	3	1–3	1.7	42.0	10	4.36	_____	___/___
2	2	4–5	3	80.5	10	7.43	_____	___/___
3	"	6–7	4	107.3	10	9.58	_____	___/___
4	3	8–10	5	134.1	10	11.73	_____	___/___
5	2	11–12	"	"	15	15.18	_____	___/___
6	3	13–14	6	160.9	15	18.01	_____	___/___
Recovery		2 minutes			sitting		_____	___/___
		4 minutes			"		_____	___/___
		6 minutes			"		_____	___/___
		8 minutes			"		_____	___/___

Comments:

*Adapted from Ellestad, M. H.: *Stress Testing. Principles and Practice.* Philadelphia: F. A.
Davis Co., 1975.

*Kattus Treadmill Test**

I. Preliminary Data   Subject＿＿＿＿＿＿＿＿＿＿＿＿＿＿＿＿＿＿＿
    Resting Heart Rate ＿＿＿＿   Resting Blood Pressure ＿＿/＿＿
    Age ＿＿＿＿   Test Administrator(s)＿＿＿＿＿＿＿＿＿＿＿＿＿＿＿＿＿＿＿

II. Graded Exercise Test

Stage	Duration (minutes)	Time (minutes)	Speed (mph & m/min)		Grade (%)	Mets	Heart Rate	Blood Pressure
1	3	1–3	1.5	40.2	10	4.22	＿＿＿	＿＿/＿＿
2	"	4–6	2.0	53.6	10	5.29	＿＿＿	＿＿/＿＿
3	"	7–9	2.5	67.0	10	6.36	＿＿＿	＿＿/＿＿
4	"	10–12	3.0	80.5	10	7.43	＿＿＿	＿＿/＿＿
5	"	13–15	3.5	93.8	10	8.5	＿＿＿	＿＿/＿＿
6	"	16–19	4.0	107.3	10	9.58	＿＿＿	＿＿/＿＿

END OF SUBMAX. EXERCISE

Stage	Duration (minutes)	Time (minutes)	Speed (mph & m/min)		Grade (%)	Mets	Heart Rate	Blood Pressure
7	"	20–23	"	"	14	11.79	＿＿＿	＿＿/＿＿
8	"	24–27	"	"	18	14	＿＿＿	＿＿/＿＿
9	"	28–31	"	"	22	16.2	＿＿＿	＿＿/＿＿

Recovery							
	2 minutes		sitting	＿＿＿	＿＿＿
	4 minutes		"	＿＿＿	＿＿/＿＿
	6 minutes		"	＿＿＿	＿＿/＿＿
	8 minutes		"	＿＿＿	＿＿/＿＿

Comments:

*Adapted from Kattus, A. A.: Physical training and heteradrenergic blocking drugs in modifying coronary insufficiency. *In* Marchetti, G. and B. Toccardi (eds): *Coronary Circulation and Energetics of the Myocardium.* New York: Karger, 1967.

*Naughton Treadmill Test**

I. Preliminary Data   Subject_____ _____
    Resting Heart Rate _____ Resting Blood Pressure _____
    Age _____   Test Administrator(s)_____
II. Graded Exercise Test

Stage	Duration (minutes)	Time (minutes)	Speed (mph & m/min)		Grade (%)	Mets	Heart Rate	Blood Pressure
1	2	1–2	1	26.8	0	1.77	_____	___/___
2	"	3–4	2.0	53.6	0	2.53	_____	___/___
3	"	5–6	"	"	3.5	3.5	_____	___/___
4	"	7–8	"	"	7.0	4.46	_____	___/___
5	"	9–10	"	"	10.5	5.43	_____	___/___
6	"	11–12	"	"	14	6.39	_____	___/___
7	"	13–14	"	"	17.5	7.36	_____	___/___
Recovery		2 minutes			sitting		_____	___/___
		4 minutes			"		_____	___/___
		6 minutes			"		_____	___/___
		8 minutes			"		_____	___/___

Comments:

*Adapted from Naughton, J., B. Balke, and F. Nagle: Refinements in methods of evaluation and physical conditioning before and after myocardial infarction. *Am. J. Cardiol.* 14:837, 1964.

Wilson (Functional) Treadmill Test   *(Beginning)*

I. Preliminary Data   Subject_____
    Resting Heart Rate _____   Resting Blood Pressure ____/____
    Age _____   Test Administrator(s)_____
II. Graded Exercise Test

Stage	Duration (minutes)	Time (minutes)	Speed (mph & m/min)		Grade (%)	Mets	Heart Rate	Blood Pressure
1	3	1–3	1.5	40.2	0	2.15	_____	____/____
2	3	4–6	2.0	53.6	0	2.53	_____	____/____
3	3	7–9	2.5	67.0	0	2.91	_____	____/____
4	3	10–12	3.0	80.5	0	2.29	_____	____/____
5		13–15	3.0	80.5	5	5.36	_____	____/____
6		16–18	3.0	80.5	7.5	6.39	_____	____/____
7		19–21	3.0	80.5	10	7.43	_____	____/____

Recover	2 minutes	sitting	_____	_____
	minutes	"	_____	____/____
	minutes	"	_____	____/____
	8 minutes	"	_____	____/____

Comments:

Wilson (Functional) Treadmill Test   (Advanced)

I. Preliminary Data   Subject_____
    Resting Heart Rate _____ Resting Blood Pressure ____/____
    Age _____   Test Administrator(s)_____
II. Graded Exercise Test

Stage	Duration (minutes)	Time (minutes)	Speed (mph & m/min)		Grade (%)	Mets	Heart Rate	Blood Pressure
1	3	3	1.5	40.2	10	3.5	_____	____/____
2	3	6	2.0	53.6	12.5	5.38	_____	____/____
3	3	9	2.5	67.0	15	7.5	_____	____/____
4	3	12	3.0	80.5	15	9.09	_____	____/____
5	3	15	3.5	93.9	15	10.61	_____	____/____
6	3	18	4.0	107.3	15	12.12	_____	____/____
7	3	21	4.5	120.7	15	13.64	_____	____/____

Recovery								
Recovery	2 minutes				sitting		_____	____/____
	4 minutes				"		_____	____/____
	6 minutes				"		_____	____/____
	8 minutes				"		_____	____/____

Comments:

*YMCA Bicycle Test**

I. Preliminary Data   Subject_____
    Resting Heart Rate _____ Resting Blood Pressure ___/___
    Age _____   Test Administrator(s)_____
II. Exercise Test†

Stage	RPM	Workload (KPM)	Heart Rate		Blood Pressure	
1	50	300 KPM (1 Kp) (2.86 met)	_____	2nd min.	_____ /	2nd min.
			_____	3rd min.	_____ /	3rd min.
			_____		_____.___ /	
2	50	_____KPM	_____	2nd min.	_____ /	2nd min.
			_____	3rd min.	_____ /	3rd min.
			_____		_____ /	
3	50	_____KPM	_____	2nd min.	_____ /	2nd min.
			_____	3rd min.	_____ /	3rd min.
			_____		_____ /	
Recovery	2 min.		_____		_____ /	
	4 min.		_____		_____ /	
	6 min.		_____		_____ /	
	8 min.		_____		_____ /	

Comments:

*Adapted from Myers, C. R. L., Golding, A., and Sinning, W. E.: *The Y's Way to Physical Fitness*. Emmaus: Rodale Press, 1973.

†*Note*: Allow the subject to work at first workload for three minutes. Count the heart rate at the last half of the second and third minutes. If heart rates in the second and third minutes differ by more than 5 beats/min., extend the ride for an extra minute or until this stable value is obtained. According to the heart rate attained at the last minute of the first workload move to the second workload, and then, accordingly, to the third workload. Endpoint: reaching a pre-set submaximal heart rate level.

Equipment and Supply Companies

Abbott Medical Electronics Co.
Dept. 700, AP 14
Abbott Park
North Chicago, Illinois   60064

Aerobics, Inc.
Clifton, New Jersey   07013

American Hospital Supply
General Office 1450
Wauketan Road
McGaw Park, Illinois   60085

American Optical Medical Division
P.O. Box 361
Bedford, Massachusetts   01730

Avionics Biomedical Division
6901 West Imperial Highway
Los Angeles, California   90045

Battle Creek Equipment Co.
307 West Jackson Street
Battle Creek, Michigan   49017

Baum Instruments
620 Oak Street
Coiaque, New York   11726

Beckman Instruments, Inc.
P.O. Box 66204
Chicago, Illinois   60666

248

Birtcher Corporation
4371 Valley Blvd.
Los Angeles, California   90032

Burdick Corporation
13755 Fordham Court
Applevalley, Minnesota   55124

Cambridge Instrument Company
73 Spring Street
Ossining, New York   10562

Collins Company
220 Wood Road
Braintree, Massachusetts   02184

Datascope Corporation
520 Victor Street
Saddle Brook, New Jersey   07662

D & D Medical
830 E. Armour Road
Oconomowoc, Wisconsin   53066

The Dann Company
24300 High Point Road
Beachwood, Ohio   44122

Elmed Incorporated
60 West Fay Avenue
Addison, Illinois   60101

Electrodyne Division of Becton, Dickinson & Co.
Sharon, Massachusetts   12167

Electronics for Medicine, Inc.
30 Virginia Road
White Plains, New York   10603

Electro-Technics, Inc.
622 Cascade Road
Pittsburgh, Pennsylvania   15221

Fitness Industries
P.O. Box 448
Pelham, Alabama   35124

Fukuda Denshi Co., Ltd.
3-30-4
Hongo, Bunkyo-Ku
Toyko 113, Japan

General Electric Company
Medical Systems Division
4855 Electric Avenue
Milwaukee, Wisconsin   53201

Gilson Medical Electronics, Inc.
P.O. Box 27
Middleton, Wisconsin   53562

Gould Inc.
Instruments Systems Division
3631 Perkins Avenue
Cleveland, Ohio   44114

Harvard Apparatus Co., Inc.
150 North Dover Road
Millis, Massachusetts   02054

Hewlett Packard
2400 N. Prior
Roseville, Minnesota   55113

Instrumentation Laboratory, Inc.
Lexington, Massachusetts   02173

International Medical Corporation
One Inverness Drive East
Englewood, Colorado   80110

IPCO Hospital Supply Corporation
1025 Westchester Avenue
White Plains, New York   10604

Irex Medical Systems, Inc.
109 Croton Avenue
Ossining, New York   10562

James Phillips Company
10208 Union Terrace Lane
Maple Grove, Minnesota   55369

Labarge, Inc.
16952 Old Elm Drive
Country Club Hills, Illinois   60477

Lafayette Instrument Co.
Box 1279
LaFayette, Indiana   47902

LaRoche Medical Electronics Division
Hoffmann-La Roche Inc.
Cranbury, New Jersey   08512

Litton Medical Products, Inc.
Medical Electronics
825 Nicholas Blvd.
Elk Grove, Illinois   60007

Lumex, Inc.
Cyben Division
100 Spence Street
Bay Shore, New York   11706

MacLevy Products Corp.
92–21 Corona Avenue
Elmhurst, New York   11373

Marquette Electronics, Inc.
8200 West Tower Avenue
Milwaukee, Wisconsin   53223

Medcraft Incorporated
Box 542
Skippack, Pennsylvania   19474

Med Data, Inc.
P.O. Box 4423
2304 University Avenue
Madison, Wisconsin   53711

Medical Electronics
436 N. Clark Street
Chicago, Illinois   60610

Medical Research Laboratories
1873 Busse Highway
Des Plaines, Illinois   60016

Medrad
4084 Mt. Royal Boulevard
Allison Park, Pa.   15101

Mid-West Instrument Co.
2520 Lyndale Avenue, South
Minneapolis, Minnesota   55401

Modern Dynamics
1538 College
South Houston, Texas   77587

Narco Bio-Systems, Inc.
7651 Airport Blvd.
P.O. Box 12522
Houston, Texas   77017

New Dimensions in Medicine
3040 East River Road
Dayton, Ohio   45439

Owl Instruments Ltd.
61 Alness Street
Downsview, Ontario
Canada M3J 2H2

Paramount Health Equipment Corp.
3000 S. Santa Fe Ave.
Los Angeles, CA   90058

Parke, Davis and Company
Medical Instruments Division
180 Bear Hill Road
Waltham, Massachusetts   02154

Pioneer Medical Systems, Inc.
321 Ellis Street
New Britain, Connecticut   06051

Physio-Control Corporation
11811 Willows Road
Redmond, Washington   98052

Physiological Data Systems
Honeywell Test Instruments Division
P.O. Box 5227
Denver, Colorado   80217

Pride Co. Inc.
Box 225
Huntington, Indiana   46750

Quinton Instruments
3051—44th Avenue West
Seattle, Washington   98199

Seimens Corporation
5501 West State Street
Milwaukee, Wisconsin   53208

Sierra Medical Sales
P.O. Box 4248
Riverside, California   92504

Stratham Instruments, Inc.
2230 Stratham Blvd.
Oxnard, California   93030

Taylor Corporation
112 North Oak Park Avenue
Oak Park, Illinois   60301

Tektronix, Inc.
P.O. Box 500
Beaverton, Oregon   67077

Tingle Athletic Equipment Inc.
Route 4, Box 359
Houston, Texas   77036

Trotter Treadmills
95 Marked Tree Rd.
Holliston, Massachusetts   01746

appendix **F**

Summary of the La Crosse Cardiac Rehabilitation Program

Figure A is an organizational chart of the La Crosse Cardiac Rehabilitation program, indicating the patient population comprising each phase, the duration of each phase, and the type of graded exercise test (GXT) conducted in each phase. The patient population of Phase I consists of those with unstable angina pectoris or those convalescing from either a myocardial infarction or cardiac surgery. This in-patient phase normally lasts 14 to 17 days, and concludes with a submaximal, low-exertion discharge graded exercise test (DiGXT).

Phase II is a multifaceted approach to rehabilitation that allows diverse means to meet the unique needs and interests of the patient. The patient may elect a "home" program consisting of walking or using a stationary bicycle ergometer, or may wish to participate in an out-patient clinic program involving ECG-telemetered exercise on such devices as a bicycle ergometer, treadmill, rowing machine, steps, or arm wheel. Regardless of the exercise mode chosen, patients in Phase II periodically receive an exercise prescription check involving ECG monitored exercise. The prescription check is to review symptoms and medication effect, and to adjust the exercise prescription. Cardiac patients who have progressed from Phase I, those who are considered "highly prone" to CAD, and documented CAD patients may

252

participate in Phase II. After concluding Phase II, which usually lasts two months, the patient receives a symptom-limited maximal graded exercise test (SL-Max GXT) to evaluate maximal functional capacity, and to develop an exercise prescription for Phase III.

Patients who progress through Phase II, as well as stable cardiac patients and those prone to CAD, may elect to continue their rehabilitation efforts by becoming participants in the Phase III "maintenance" program. Again the individual may participate on an individual basis at home, utilizing walking or an indoor stationary mode of exercise, or may elect to participate in a group program involving swimming, cycling, walking or jogging, which is conducted at a local community service agency such as a YMCA, elementary school facility, or a university facility. Entrance to Phase III requires a symptom-limited maximal GXT followed by the development of an exercise prescription. Follow-up exercising and exercise prescription checks are routine as the patient continues in Phase III.

Fig. A

CARDIAC REHABILITATION PROGRAM
GUNDERSEN CLINIC, LTD. & LA CROSSE EXERCISE PROGRAM (UW-L)
La Crosse, Wisconsin

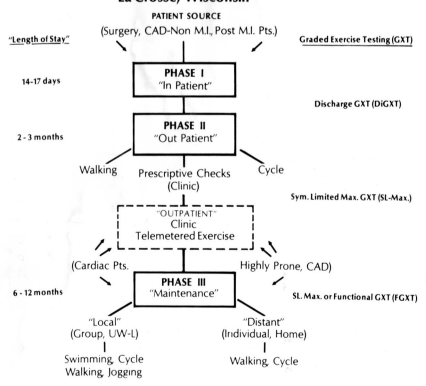